I. Jon Russell, MD, PhD
Editor

The Fibromyalgia Syndrome: A Clinical Case Definition for Practitioners

The Fibromyalgia Syndrome: A Clinical Case Definition for Practitioners has been co-published simultaneously as *Journal of Musculoskeletal Pain*, Volume 11, Number 4 2003.

Pre-publication
REVIEWS,
COMMENTARIES,
EVALUATIONS . . .

"A MONUMENTAL WORK! For the first time, a single text documents signs and symptoms, pathophysiology, physical evaluation, and treatment–all the fine points–that were previously known by only a few skilled specialists. Other physicians have frequently asked me, 'Is there a reliable and authoritative text dealing with Fibromyalgia Syndrome?' Until now I could offer none. This text is an exhaustive and all-encompassing work that WILL HELP ANY PRACTITIONER TO BETTER UNDERSTAND AND MANAGE FIBROMYALGIA. I will recommend it to all my colleagues!"

Charles W. Lapp, MD
Director
Hunter-Hopkins Center
Assistant Consulting Professor
Duke University Medical Center

More pre-publication
REVIEWS, COMMENTARIES, EVALUATIONS . . .

"I highly recommend this COMPREHENSIVE, WELL-REFERENCED, AND PRACTICAL TEXT as a required resource for healthcare professionals and patients alike. This work provides a scientifically and clinically sound framework for further study in the field of fibromyalgia. Prepared by well-regarded authorities, the statements and reviews on the levels of evidence that support proposed treatments and casual factors are particularly informative."

Roberto Patarca-Montero, MD, PhD, HCLD
Member
Chronic Fatigue Syndrome Advisory Committee
to the US Secretary of Health
Chairman
Education Subcommittee

"REALLY USEFUL, NOT ONLY FOR PHYSICIANS, BUT ALSO FOR PATIENTS. This book is AN EXCITING CONSENSUS DOCUMENT based on a meeting of an expert subcommittee of Health Canada. It deals with the clinical definition, diagnosis, treatment, and international research activities related to the Fibromyalgia Syndrome. In my opinion it should become a bestseller in this field."

Dieter Pongratz, Dr. Med.
Professor
Department of Neurology
University of Munich Hospital
Friedrich Baur Institute
Munich, Germany

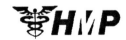

The Haworth Medical Press
An Imprint of The Haworth Press, Inc.

The Fibromyalgia Syndrome:
A Clinical Case Definition
for Practitioners

The Fibromyalgia Syndrome: A Clinical Case Definition for Practitioners has been co-published simultaneously as *Journal of Musculoskeletal Pain*, Volume 11, Number 4 2003.

The *Journal of Musculoskeletal Pain* Monographic "Separates"

Below is a list of "separates," which in serials librarianship means a special issue simultaneously published as a special journal issue or double-issue *and* as a "separate" hardbound monograph. [This is a format which we also call a "DocuSerial."]

"Separates" are published because specialized libraries or professionals may wish to purchase a specific thematic issue by itself in a format which can be separately cataloged and shelved, as opposed to purchasing the journal on an on-going basis. Faculty members may also more easily consider a "separate" for classroom adoption.

"Separates" are carefully classified separately with the major book jobbers so that the journal tie-in can be noted on new book order slips to avoid duplicate purchasing.

You may wish to visit Haworth's website at . . .

http://www.HaworthPress.com

. . . to search our online catalog for complete tables of contents of these separates and related publications.

You may also call 1-800-HAWORTH [outside US/Canada: 607-722-5857], or Fax 1-800-895-0582 [outside US/Canada: 607-771-0012], or e-mail at:

docdelivery@haworthpress.com

The Fibromyalgia Syndrome: A Clinical Case Definition for Practitioners, edited by I. Jon Russell, MD, PhD (Vol. 11, No. 4, 2003). *Establishes an expert consensus toward a working case definition of fibromyalgia syndrome and a working guide to its management for physicians in Canada.*

The Clinical Neurobiology of Fibromyalgia and Myofascial Pain: Therapeutic Implications, edited by Robert M. Bennett, MD (Vol. 10, No. 1/2, 2002). *Covers the latest developments in pain research: examines the results of a wide scope of basic and applied research on soft-tissue pain.*

International MYOPAIN Society–MYOPAIN '01: Abstracts from the 5th World Congress on Myofascial Pain and Fibromyalgia, Portland, Oregon, USA, September 9-September 13, 2001 (Vol. 9, Suppl. #5, 2001)

Muscle Pain, Myofascial Pain, and Fibromyalgia: Recent Advances, edited by Leonardo Vecchiet, MD, and Maria Adele Giamberardino, MD (Vol. 7, No. 1/2, 1999). *Covers the latest developments in musculoskeletal pain that were presented at the MYOPAIN '98 Congress in Silvi Marina, Italy.*

MYOPAIN '98: Abstracts from the 4th World Congress on Myofascial Pain and Fibromyalgia, Silvi Marina [TE], ITALY, August 24-August 27, 1998, edited by Leonardo Vecchiet, MD, and Maria Adele Giamberardino, MD (Vol. 6, Supp. #2, 1998).

The Neuroscience and Endocrinology of Fibromyalgia, edited by Stanley R. Pillemer, MD (Vol. 6, No. 3, 1998). *"I recommend this book to all health care providers who want to offer the most up-to-date therapy for their patients with fibromyalgia." [David Borestein, MD, Clinical Professor of Medicine, The George Washington University Medical Center, Arthritis and Rheumatism]*

Muscle Pain Syndromes and Fibromyalgia: Pressure Algometry for Quantification of Diagnosis and Treatment Outcome, edited by Andrew A. Fischer, MD, PhD (Vol. 6, No. 1, 1998). *"Should help researchers in developing new and expanded studies for the appropriate role of pressure algometry." [Martin Grabois, MD, Professor and Chairman, Physical Medicine and Rehabilitation, Baylor College of Medicine, Houston, Texas]*

Musculoskeletal Pain Emanating from the Head and Neck: Current Concepts in Diagnosis, Management, and Cost Containment, edited by Murray E. Allen, MD (Vol. 4, No. 4, 1996). *"Exciting because it contains a distillation of recent research that is of value to all who treat and serve those with whiplash-related injuries." [National Association of Rehabilitation Professionals in the Private Sector]*

Clinical Overview and Pathogenesis of the Fibromyalgia Syndrome, Myofascial Pain Syndrome, and Other Pain Syndromes, edited by I. Jon Russell, MD, PhD (Vol. 4, No. 1/2, 1996). *The featured speakers at the MYOPAIN '95 Third World Congress are here distilled into an anthology that represents a state of the art in fibromyalgia syndrome and myofascial pain syndrome from that conference.*

MYOPAIN '95: Abstracts from the 3rd World Congress on Myofascial Pain and Fibromyalgia, San Antonio, Texas, USA, July 30-August 3, 1995, edited by I. Jon Russell, MD, PhD (Vol. 3, Supp. #1, 1995). *An excellent resource that allows physicians, dentists, researchers, and others working in this field to access key information as presented by specialists worldwide who work with and research chronic muscle pain.*

Fibromyalgia, Chronic Fatigue Syndrome, and Repetitive Strain Injury: Current Concepts in Diagnosis, Management, Disability, and Health Economics, edited by Andrew Chalmers, MD, Geoffrey Owen Littlejohn, MD, Irving Salit, MD, and Frederick Wolfe, MD (Vol. 3, No. 2, 1995). *"The information and original research presented is relevant and useful for understanding some of the global research being conducted on these disorders. . . . It would be most useful as an addition to a scientific/medical library." [Annals of Pharmacotherapy]*

The Fibromyalgia Syndrome: Current Research and Future Directions in Epidemiology, Pathogenesis, and Treatment, edited by Stanley R. Pillemer, MD (Vol. 2, No. 3, 1994). *"This highly informative and well-referenced text is recommended to both students and practitioners." [Annals of Pharmacotherapy]*

Musculoskeletal Pain, Myofascial Pain Syndrome, and the Fibromyalgia Syndrome: Proceedings from the Second World Congress on Myofascial Pain and Fibromyalgia, edited by Søren Jacobsen, MD, Bente Danneskiold-Samsøe, MD, PhD, and Birger Lund, MD, PhD (Vol. 1, No. 3/4, 1993). *"Packed with state-of-the-art information. . . . An important contribution to our understanding of myofascial pain syndrome, fibromyalgia, and musculoskeletal pain, and will be useful to both patients and health care providers." [Lifeline [National Chronic Pain Outreach Association]]*

The Fibromyalgia Syndrome:
A Clinical Case Definition
for Practitioners

I. Jon Russell, MD, PhD

Editor

The Fibromyalgia Syndrome: A Clinical Case Definition for Practitioners has been co-published simultaneously as *Journal of Musculoskeletal Pain*, Volume 11, Number 4 2003.

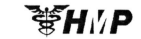

The Haworth Medical Press®
An Imprint of The Haworth Press, Inc.

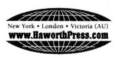

New York • London • Victoria (AU)
www.HaworthPress.com

Published by

The Haworth Medical Press®, 10 Alice Street, Binghamton, NY 13904-1580 USA

The Haworth Medical Press® is an imprint of The Haworth Press, Inc., 10 Alice Street, Binghamton, NY 13904-1580 USA.

The Fibromyalgia Syndrome: A Clinical Case Definition for Practitioners has been co-published simultaneously as *Journal of Musculoskeletal Pain*, Volume 11, Number 4 2003.

Cover design by Marylouise E. Doyle

Library of Congress Cataloging-in-Publication Data

The fibromyalgia syndrome : a clinical case definition for practitioners / I. Jon Russell, editor.
     p. ; cm. – (Journal of musculoskeletal pain, ISSN 1058-2452 ; v. 11, no. 4)
    Includes bibliographical references and index.
    ISBN 0-7890-2574-4 (soft cover : alk. paper)
    1. Fibromyalgia.
    [DNLM: 1. Fibromyalgia–diagnosis. 2. Clinical Protocols. 3. Diagnosis, Differential. 4. Fibromyalgia–therapy. WE 544 F4418
2004] I. Russell, I. Jon. II. Series.
RC927.3F526 2004
616.7'42–dc22
                                                      2004004109

Indexing, Abstracting & Website/Internet Coverage

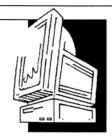

Journal of Musculoskeletal Pain

This section provides you with a list of major indexing & abstracting services. That is to say, each service began covering this periodical during the year noted in the right column. Most Websites which are listed below have indicated that they will either post, disseminate, compile, archive, cite, or alert their own Website users with research-based content from this work. [This list is as current as the copyright date of this publication.]

Abstracting, Website/Indexing Coverage ....Year When Coverage Began

- *AnalgesiaFile, Dannemiller Memorial Educational Foundation, Texas*
  <http://www.pain.com>.. 2003

- *Behavioral Medicine Abstracts* 1994

- *Biology Digest [in print & online]*................................... 2000

- *Cambridge Scientific Abstracts [Calcium & Calcified Tissue Abstracts/Health & Safety*
  Science Abstracts] <http://www.csa.com> 1993

- *Centre Regional D'Exploration des Myalgies <http://www.infomyalgie.com>* 1996

- *CFS-NEWS* 1999

- *CINAHL [Cumulative Index to Nursing & Allied Health Literature], in print, EBSCO,*
  and SilverPlatter, Data-Star, and PaperChase. [Support materials include Subject
  Heading List, Database Search Guide, and instructional video]
  <http://www.cinahl.com> 1995

- *CNPIEC Reference Guide: Chinese National Directory of Foreign Periodicals* 1995

- *Current Contents/Clinical Medicine <http://www.isinet.com>* 1997

- *EMBASE/Excerpta Medica Secondary Publishing Division <http://www.elsevier.nl>*....... 1993

- *e-psyche, LLC <http://www.e-psyche.net>* 2001

- *Environmental Sciences and Pollution Management [Cambridge Scientific Abstracts*
  Internet Database Service] <http://www.csa.com> .... *

- *Ergonomics Abstracts* 1993

- *Excerpta Medica . . . See EMBASE/Excerpta Medica* 1993

- *FM Forum British Columbia Fibromyalgia Society* 1996

- *Health & Psychosocial Instruments [HaPI] Database [available through online*
  and as a CD-ROM from Ovid Technologies]................................. 2002

- *Industrial Hygiene Digest* 1996

- *ISI Web of Science <http://www.isinet.com>* 2003

[continued]

* Exact start date to come.

Special Bibliographic Notes related to special journal issues [separates] and indexing/abstracting:

- indexing/abstracting services in this list will also cover material in any "separate" that is co-published simultaneously with Haworth's special thematic journal issue or DocuSerial. Indexing/abstracting usually covers material at the article/chapter level.
- monographic co-editions are intended for either non-subscribers or libraries which intend to purchase a second copy for their circulating collections.
- monographic co-editions are reported to all jobbers/wholesalers/approval plans. The source journal is listed as the "series" to assist the prevention of duplicate purchasing in the same manner utilized for books-in-series.
- to facilitate user/access services all indexing/abstracting services are encouraged to utilize the co-indexing entry note indicated at the bottom of the first page of each article/chapter/contribution.
- this is intended to assist a library user of any reference tool [whether print, electronic, online, or CD-ROM] to locate the monographic version if the library has purchased this version but not a subscription to the source journal.
- individual articles/chapters in any Haworth publication are also available through the Haworth Document Delivery Service [HDDS].

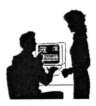

The Fibromyalgia Syndrome:
A Clinical Case Definition
for Practitioners

CONTENTS

ABOUT THE EDITOR

I. Jon Russell, MD, PhD, is Associate Professor of Medicine at The University of Texas Health Science Center in San Antonio, where he is also Director of the University Clinical Research Center. He is the founding Editor of the *Journal of Musculoskeletal Pain* and has guided its progress since 1993. He was Founding President of the International MYOPAIN Society and currently serves as a Board Member of that organization. He is a member of the Editorial Board of *Pain Watch*. Dr. Russell is an internationally recognized researcher and clinical practitioner caring for patients with a wide variety of musculoskeletal pain disorders but with emphasis on the fibromyalgia syndrome. He serves on expert panels for fibromyalgia syndrome support organizations in the United States, Canada, and France.

Dr. Russell has twice been the National Chairman for the American College of Rheumatology's Nonarticular Rheumatism Study Group and has been a Counselor for the Central Region of the American College of Rheumatology. He has served on the Research Grants Committee for the Arthritis Foundation and on the Research and Development Grants Committee of the Audie Murphy Veterans Administration Hospital.

Dr. Russell has been honored by listings in *The Best Doctors in America, The Best Doctors in America: Central Region, The Best Doctors in the South and Southwest*, and *The Best 2000 Doctors in America*. His service to the South Texas community was acknowledged with the Humanitarian of the Year Award [1994] by the South Central Texas Chapter of the Arthritis Foundation.

Dr. Russell is the author of over 85 original publications and over 30 chapters in medical textbooks. He is co-author of *The Fibromyalgia Help Book*, and producer of the video documentary "Fibromyalgia and You," two educational resources for people with fibromyalgia. He travels extensively, speaking to medical and lay audiences about musculoskeletal pain and medical education issues. With a doctorate in biochemistry and nutrition, a medical degree, residency in internal medicine, subspecialty in rheumatology, 25 years of pain research, and an experienced world view, Dr. Russell brings to this journal an interdisciplinary perspective and background to emerging issues in both research and clinical practice.

Preface:
Back to the Future

This entire special issue of the *Journal of Musculoskeletal Pain* [*JMP*] is devoted to presentation of what will likely to be called the Canadian Consensus Document on Fibromyalgia Syndrome [FMS] (1). The document encompasses a very broad scope, involving a clinical case definition, diagnosis, and management of FMS. In addition, the importance of research findings within the FMS construct has prompted the inclusion of a section regarding what is known about the pathogenesis of FMS. The history of the development of this document, which was supported by Health Canada, is outlined in a companion editorial (2) by its physician editors and the lay group coordinator of the project.

The clinical case definition proposed by the Expert Consensus Panel (1) chosen by Health Canada is based on the reasonable judgment of Panel members who have considerable experience with FMS in academic and community environments. In the same way that the Delphi of the 1990 ACR Criteria study were properly entrusted to know the disorder based on their extensive clinical experience, so the Panel members, in their composite wisdom, were considered to perceive what was likely to prove to be useful in the community.

This undertaking can be viewed as a the next step in a long-term plan. Since the development of the American College of Rheumatology [ACR] 1990 Classification Criteria for the Fibromyalgia Syndrome (3), it has been clear that eventually it would be necessary to determine what to include in a clinical case definition for use in community medicine. The ACR Criteria were developed to guide the uniform selection of FMS patients for entry into research studies. The ACR Criteria have made it possible for a reader of FMS research to have confidence that studies done separately in Wichita, Peoria, Boston, Portland, and San Antonio were evaluating comparable patients. The same applies to studies performed in Europe and Asia that have espoused the ACR Criteria. On the other hand, there has been no certainty that the 1990 ACR Criteria would properly identify all of the affected individuals in a community clinic while properly excluding those who should not be given this diagnosis.

The 1990 ACR Criteria utilized statistical analysis to establish a somewhat arbitrary cut in the number [at least 11 affected of 18 anatomically-named] of body sites, called tender points [TePs], that were unusually sensitive to deep digital palpation pressure and were required for a patient to enter a FMS research study. That was a reasonable approach to standardizing enrollment in pivotal research about a Delphi-defined disorder. On the other hand, some (4) have argued that it is improper to use the 1990 ACR criteria for diagnosis in community medical practice. Of course, physicians in clinical practice have applied the 1990 ACR criteria diagnostically because body pain is such a major clinical problem and there is nothing more precise than the 1990 ACR Criteria for identifying patients with FMS. Nothing comparable has been created and or validated for use in community medicine. Frankly, the only reason anyone really cares what physicians diagnose in the confines of their practices is that the diagnosis of FMS can then take on legal [compensation] implications for which someone has to pay. Another view, with similar implications, holds that management strategies [often expensive ones] found to work for FMS should be made available to community patients with ten or less TePs, especially if they have typical FMS associated symptoms, such as chronic insomnia, prolonged morning stiffness, or irritable bowel syndrome.

The development of the Canadian Clinical Case Definition for FMS can be viewed as the first concerted effort to correct this deficit. It is hoped that the process of validation will eventually benefit both the practitioners and their patients.

The clinical case definition proposed in the Canadian Consensus Document (1) contains elements very similar to those proposed by Yunus and coworkers in 1989 (5), hence the title of the Preface, "Back to the Future." While new, this approach to the diagnosis and management of FMS uses what has been learned about FMS since 1990 and addresses previously expressed concerns. Thus, clinicians have recognized that patients who met the 1990 ACR Criteria for Classification of FMS can also exhibit a variety of clinical manifestations other than body pain and tenderness, such as insomnia, cognitive complaints, headaches, morning stiffness, and affective symptoms. Those concerns have also been the basis for many of the pharmaceutical based studies involving FMS patients. The main objective of the Canadian Consensus Document (1) is to enhance the ability of Canadian community physicians to recognize and treat FMS in their practices and to be more aware of its many clinical manifestations, including pain, and beyond. The extent to which its influence extends beyond Canada is yet to be seen.

This document addresses previous concerns and presents a clinical case definition that the international scientific community can refine as needed and then should attempt to validate. To facilitate that process, the *JMP* editorial staff have contacted two well-respected epidemiologists, with established track records in studying FMS. Each was asked to apply established epidemiological and statistical methods in the design of a study to validate a clinical case definition for use in community medicine. The Research Ideas section of this volume provides three short manuscripts. The first (6)

is a summary of the challenge given to the epidemiologists. That is followed by outlines from each of the experts (7,8) indicating what needs to be done and how it could be accomplished using the Canadian Consensus Document (1) as a resource. These efforts will help to resolve conceptual, legal, and other disputes that have arisen from the clinical application of the 1990 ACR Criteria Research Definition for FMS.

The panel had no illusion that everyone in the field would be completely satisfied with the document as it now stands. The proposed Canadian Clinical Case Definition must be submitted to further research scrutiny in the relevant settings. The definitive study will be expensive. It must be carefully planned by those with much experience in this process. It will require international cooperation between interested parties from a variety of disciplines and holding different views. The main requirements for professional participation in the proposed study should be a willingness to contribute selflessly to the effort and a commitment to accept the scientific outcome. Strong advocacy will be needed to develop an airtight protocol and to secure adequate funding to do the job right. It is expected that there will be honest disagreements that must be amicably negotiated, but cynical detractors and bodacious naysayers must be ignored. The readers of *JMP* are invited to voice opinions in the form of Letters to the Editor.

I. Jon Russell, MD, PhD
The Editor

REFERENCES

1. Jain AK, Carruthers BM, van de Sande MI, Barron SR, Donaldson CCS, Dunne JV, Gingrich E, Heffez DS, Leung FY-K, Malone DJ, Romano TJ, Russell IJ, Saul D, Seibel DG: Fibromyalgia syndrome: Canadian clinical working case definition, diagnostic and treatment protocols–a consensus document. J Musculoske Pain 11(4):3-107, 2003.

2. Jain AK, Carruthers BM, van de Sande MI: Introduction: Canadian Consensus Document on Fibromyalgia Syndrome. J Musculoske Pain 11(4):1-2, 2003.

3. Wolfe F, Smythe HA, Yunus MB, Bennett RM, Bombardier C, Goldenberg DL, Tugwell P, Campbell SM, Abeles M, Clark P, Fam AG, Farber SJ, Fiechtner JJ, Franklin CM, Gatter RA, Hamaty D, Lessard J, Lichtbroun AS, Masi AT, McCain GA, Reynolds WJ,

Romano TJ, Russell IJ, Sheon RP: The American College of Rheumatology 1990 Criteria for the Classification of Fibromyalgia. Arthritis Rheum 33:160-172, 1990.

4. Wolfe F: Stop using the American College of Rheumatology Criteria in the clinic. J Rheumatol 30(8): 1671-1672, 2003.

5. Yunus MB, Masi AT, Aldag JC: Preliminary criteria for primary fibromyalgia syndrome (PFS): Multivariate analysis of a consecutive series of PFS, other pain patients, and normal subjects. Clin Exp Rheumatol 7:63-69, 1989.

6. Russell IJ: Proposed study to develop and validate a clinical case definition for the fibromyalgia syndrome applicable to the community practice setting. J Musculoske Pain 11(4):109-111, 2003.

7. White KP: Developing and validating a clinical case definition for the fibromyalgia syndrome for use in clinical practice. J Musculoske Pain 11(4):117-118, 2003.

8. Raphael KG: Proposed methods for validation of a clinical case definition of the fibromyalgia syndrome. J Musculoske Pain 11(4):113-115, 2003.

Introduction:
Canadian Consensus Document
on Fibromyalgia Syndrome

The National ME/FM Action Network [Canada] spearheaded the drive for the development of an expert consensus document, which would include a clinical definition, diagnostic and treatment protocols, and a discussion of pertinent research for the Fibromyalgia Syndrome [FMS]. As increasing numbers of FMS patients asked about knowledgeable doctors, it quickly became clear that there was a need for more education about FMS among primary care practitioners. The Network sent out a questionnaire to doctors across Canada asking what items would be most helpful in assisting them with their FMS patients. The physicians concurred that a clinical definition, as well as diagnostic and treatment protocols, were of prime importance.

The National ME/FM Action Network then approached two clinicians knowledgeable and experienced in FMS, Dr. Anil Jain of Ontario and Dr. Bruce Carruthers of British Columbia, who agreed to co-author a draft document. Lydia Neilson, President of the National ME/FM Action Network, met with the Honourable Alan Rock, then Minister of Health, to discuss the results of the doctors' survey and the draft document. The Honourable Alan Rock responded by stating the draft clinical definition was "a milestone in the fight against this complex and tragic condition."

Health Canada set up an expert medical subcommittee, which established the "Terms of Reference" for the consensus panel. One of the stipulations was that at least one member of the panel must be nominated by each of the five stakeholder groups of government, universities, clinicians, industry, and advocacy. There were to be at least ten members on the panel, four of whom could come from outside of Canada. The members of the panel must be either practicing MDs, actively treating and/or diagnosing FMS, or MDs or PhDs involved in clinical research of the illness. The focus was to provide the generalist with a clinical definition that addressed a broader spectrum of the pathogenesis of the illness, as well as provide diagnostic and treatment protocols. The panel would have autonomy over their consensus document.

The expert medical subcommittee of Health Canada selected an expert consensus panel for FMS, which consisted of thirteen members. This thirteen-member consensus panel had received a total of forty-six nominations, which included numerous nominations from each stakeholder group. The members of the consensus panel represented clinicians, university medical faculty, and researchers in the area of FMS. Collectively, they had diagnosed and/or treated more than twenty thousand FMS patients.

Health Canada planned for a Consensus Workshop to be held on March 30 to April 1, 2001. All members of the expert consensus panel were sent the draft document, which

[Haworth co-indexing entry note]: "Introduction: Canadian Consensus Document on Fibromyalgia Syndrome." Jain, Anil Kumar, Bruce M. Carruthers, and Marjorie I. van de Sande. Co-published simultaneously in *Journal of Musculoskeletal Pain* [The Haworth Medical Press, an imprint of The Haworth Press, Inc.] Vol. 11, No. 4, 2003, pp. 1-2; and: *The Fibromyalgia Syndrome: A Clinical Case Definition for Practitioners* [ed: I. Jon Russell] The Haworth Medical Press, an imprint of The Haworth Press, Inc., 2003, pp. 1-2. Single or multiple copies of this article are available for a fee from The Haworth Document Delivery Service [1-800-HAWORTH, 9:00 a.m. - 5:00 p.m. [EST]. E-mail address: docdelivery@haworthpress.com].

http://www.haworthpress.com/web/JMP
Digital Object Identifer: 10.1300/J094v11n04_01

went through three rounds of revision prior to the Consensus Workshop.

Crystaal [Biovail Pharmaceuticals] kindly agreed to fund the workshop without having any direct involvement or any financial interest in the outcome. They hired Science and Medicine Canada to organize and facilitate the workshop.

The document received consensus, in principle, at the workshop with directive for various members to revise some sections. The document was compiled by Marjorie van de Sande and sent back to the panel. There was 100% consensus by the members of the consensus panel on the final document.

Anil Kumar Jain, BSc, MD
Bruce M. Carruthers, MD, CM, FRCP[C]
Coeditors of the Consensus Document

Marjorie I. van de Sande, BEd, Grad Dip Ed
Consensus Coordinator
Director of Education
National ME/FM Action Network

ARTICLE

Fibromyalgia Syndrome:
Canadian Clinical Working Case Definition, Diagnostic and Treatment Protocols–A Consensus Document

Anil Kumar Jain
Bruce M. Carruthers
Marjorie I. van de Sande
Stephen R. Barron
C. C. Stuart Donaldson
James V. Dunne
Emerson Gingrich

Dan S. Heffez
Frances Y.-K. Leung
Daniel G. Malone
Thomas J. Romano
I. Jon Russell
David Saul
Donald G. Seibel

Anil Kumar Jain, BSc, MD, Co-Editor, is affiliated with the Ottawa Hospital, Ottawa, ON, Canada.

Bruce M. Carruthers, MD, CM, FRCP[C], Co-Editor, is Specialist in Internal Medicine, Saanichton, BC, Canada.

Marjorie I. van de Sande, BEd, Grad Dip Ed, is Consensus Coordinator, Director of Education, National ME/FM Action Network, Canada.

Stephen R. Barron, MD, CCFP, FCFP, is Clinical Assistant Professor, Department of Family Practice, Faculty of Medicine, University of British Columbia, Medical Staff, Royal Columbian Hospital, New Westminster, BC, Canada.

C. C. Stuart Donaldson, PhD, is Director of Myosymmetries, Calgary, AB, Canada.

James V. Dunne, MB, FRCP[C], is Clinical Assistant Professor, Department of Medicine, University of British Columbia, Vancouver General and St. Paul's Hospitals, Vancouver, BC, Canada.

Emerson Gingrich, MD, CCFP[C], is in Family practice, retired, Calgary, AB, Canada.

Dan S. Heffez, MD, FRCS, is President, Heffez Neurosurgical Associates S.C., and Associate Professor of Neurosurgery, Rush Medical College, Chicago, Illinois, USA.

Frances Y.-K. Leung, BSc, MD, FRCP[C], is Clinical Lecturer, Faculty of Medicine, University of Toronto, Department of Rheumatology, Sunnybrook and Women's College Health Science Centre, Department of Medicine, Saute Area Hospitals, ON, Canada.

Daniel G. Malone, MD, is Associate Professor of Medicine, University of Wisconsin, Wisconsin, USA.

Thomas J. Romano, MD, PhD, FACP, FACR, is Diplomat and President of the Board of Directors of the American Academy of Pain Management, Editorial Board and Columnist for the *Journal of Musculoskeletal Pain*, Advisory Panel, Health Points/TyH Publications, East Ohio Regional Hospital, Martins Ferry, Ohio, USA.

I. Jon Russell, MD, PhD, FACR, is Associate Professor of Medicine, Division of Clinical Immunology; Director, University Clinical Research Center, University of Texas Health Science Center, San Antonio, Texas, USA, Editor, *Journal of Musculoskeletal Pain*; International Pain Consultant to Pain Research & Management, *The Journal of the Canadian Pain Society*, London, ON; Editorial Board of *Pain Watch*, Honorary Board Member of the Lupus Foundation of America.

David Saul, MD, CCFP[C], is in Private practice, North York, ON, Canada.

Donald G. Seibel, BSc [Med], MD, CAFCI, is Medical Director, Mayfield Pain and Musculoskeletal Clinic, Edmonton, AB, Canada.

Address correspondence to: Anil K. Jain, BSc, MD, 118, 1025 Grenon Avenue, Ottawa, ON, K2B 8S5, Canada.

[Haworth co-indexing entry note]: "Fibromyalgia Syndrome: Canadian Clinical Working Case Definition, Diagnostic and Treatment Protocols–A Consensus Document." Jain, Anil Kumar et al. Co-published simultaneously in *Journal of Musculoskeletal Pain* [The Haworth Medical Press, an imprint of The Haworth Press, Inc.] Vol. 11, No. 4, 2003, pp. 3-107; and: *The Fibromyalgia Syndrome: A Clinical Case Definition for Practitioners* [ed: I. Jon Russell] The Haworth Medical Press, an imprint of The Haworth Press, Inc., 2003, pp. 3-107. Single or multiple copies of this article are available for a fee from The Haworth Document Delivery Service [1-800-HAWORTH, 9:00 a.m. - 5:00 p.m. [EST]. E-mail address: docdelivery@haworthpress.com].

http://www.haworthpress.com/web/JMP
© 2003 by The Haworth Press, Inc. All rights reserved.
Digital Object Identifer: 10.1300/J094v11n04_02

ABSTRACT. Background: There has been a growing recognition of the need for information about objective abnormalities in people with the fibromyalgia syndrome [FMS] and for an integrated approach to its diagnosis and management by primary care physicians.

Objectives: To establish an expert consensus toward a working case definition of FMS and a working guide to its management for physicians in Canada.

Methods: An Expert Subcommittee of Health Canada established the Terms of Reference and selected an Expert Medical Consensus Panel representing treating physicians, teaching faculty, and researchers. The editors prepared a draft document which was reviewed by the Panel members in preparation for the Consensus Workshop, which was held on March 30 to April 1, 2001. Subsequent writing assignments produced subdocuments on key topics relevant to the objectives. The subdocuments were then integrated into a submission document which was approved by each of the panel members.

Results: The completed document is provided. It contains sections on a new approach to case definition, on proposed research to validate the new case definition, on a practical approach to assessment of severity, on empathetic management; and on what is known about pathogenesis.

Conclusions: A consensus document was developed to assist clinicians in distinguishing FMS from other syndromes/illnesses that may present with body pain. It is intended that this document serve as a guide: to a better understanding of FMS; to a more reasoned approach to its management; and to further research on the clinical care of people with FMS. *[Article copies available for a fee from The Haworth Document Delivery Service: 1-800-HAWORTH. E-mail address: <docdelivery@haworthpress.com> Website: <http://www.HaworthPress.com> © 2003 by The Haworth Press, Inc. All rights reserved.]*

KEYWORDS. Clinical case definition, fibromyalgia syndrome, FMS, diagnostic protocol, treatment protocol, pathogenesis

INTRODUCTION

Fibromyalgia syndrome [FMS] is a chronic disorder which has been defined by a history of widespread pain and the presence of marked tenderness to palpation at standard anatomically-defined tender points (1). The World Health Organization [WHO] incorporated fibromyalgia into their 10th revision of the International Classification of Diseases [ICD] in 1991 (2). They assigned fibromyalgia number M 79.0 and classified it as a non-articular rheumatism. *Fibro* refers to fibrous tissues–ligaments and tendons, *myo* refers to muscle, and *algia* refers to pain. Distinctive reproducible pain sites called "tender points" confirm the predominant feature of widespread musculoskeletal pain. In addition to the musculoskeletal manifestations, patients commonly exhibit recurrent headaches, persistent fatigue, sleep disturbances, neurocognitive, autonomic and neuroendocrine dysfunctions, and exercise intolerance. The symptoms of FMS are prolonged, can be debilitating, and in many patients they do not resolve over time.

In 1904, Dr. William Gowers, who was mainly concerned about a form of lumbago that he considered to be different from the standard back pain, coined the term "fibrositis" to describe pain associated with fibrous or connective tissue (3). In the 1960s, the meaning of fibrositis was expanded to include diffuse musculoskeletal pain, multiple site tender points, poor sleep and fatigue (4). Heightened interest developed in the 1970s when Canadian researchers, Smythe and Moldofsky (5) demonstrated that the symptoms of fatigue and diffuse muscular pain correlated with specific changes on sleep electroencephalograms. As a result, criteria for clinical fibrositis were developed (6). Under the aegis of the American College of Rheumatology [ACR, see Appendix 1, p. 78], a large multi-center study was launched that resulted in the establishment of FMS criteria that had a clinical sensitivity of 88.4 percent and specificity of 81.1 percent. These criteria (1), which were published in 1990, have served an important function in the nosology of medicine resulting in a reliable body of comparative research data and growing recognition of fibromyalgia syndrome as a legitimate, discrete medical entity.

As the ACR definition was primarily created to *standardize research*, there has been a growing demand within the medical community for a *clinical definition*, which would be of benefit to the treating clinician. The consensus panel agreed that the ACR criteria had good sensitivity and specificity and was accepted worldwide. Based on the consensus panel's collective extensive clinical experience of diagnosing and/or treating more than twenty thousand [20,000] FMS patients, they concurred that for *clinical* purposes, it is important to include and put greater emphasis on the potential spectrum of other physiological dysfunctions, in addition to musculoskeletal pain, that can be intrinsic parts of this illness.

Our strategy for the clinical definition is to provide a flexible framework that includes the ACR criteria and encompasses more of the potential symptomatic expression of patients within the context of FMS. Grouping symptoms by shared regions of pathogenesis will enhance clarity and focus to the clinical meeting.

EPIDEMIOLOGY

A. Prevalence of FMS

The prevalence of FMS is likely underestimated as many cases are attributed to other systemic disorders or misdiagnosed as psychiatric in origin. A London, Ontario study (7) suggests that 3.3 percent of non-institutionalized adults are afflicted with FMS. Other studies suggest the prevalence is between 2 percent and 10 percent or 2,000 to 10,000 per 100,000 persons of the general population (8,9). In a prevalence study of randomly selected school children, 6.2 percent met the criteria for FMS (10). FMS is between two and five times more common than rheumatoid arthritis [RA] in the general population. As in many arthritic diseases, it predominantly affects females (8). FMS occurs most often between the ages of 35 and 50 years, but can affect all age groups.

B. Natural History of FMS

The natural history of FMS was prospectively monitored for up to eight years in a multi-center study (11). Patients completed self-assessment questionnaire forms to repeatedly quantify the severity of their pain, functional status, and affective symptoms. In general, the findings indicated that once the disorder was established, the patients continued to be

symptomatic and did not improve over that period of time. Functional disability worsened slightly.

In a follow-up study of thirty-nine patients, Kennedy and Felson found that all patients still had fibromyalgia fifteen years later. Sixty-six percent indicated that they had some improvement but 59 percent had notable fatigue, 55 percent had moderate to severe pain and/or stiffness and 48 percent had reported significant sleep difficulties (12). It should be noted that chronic sleep loss [< 7 hours per night] may shorten longevity (13).

Statistical studies estimate group prognosis. However, individual prognosis must remain a clinical estimate and is highly variable. The clinician must ascertain the severity and course of the patients' illness and impairments, as well as the patients' circumstances, environment, and the life-world to which they are responding.

C. Costs of FMS

As FMS is two to five times more common than RA (8), the approximate anticipated cost for FMS is at least double the overall direct medical cost for RA. There are important differences between FMS and RA that should be noted. Lacking the inflammation of RA, primary FMS patients are not expected to show the same degree of joint destruction and to require the very costly total joint arthroplasties that are often needed by the RA patient with aggressive erosive disease.

Evidence from a multi-center study conducted in the United States (14) and a single center study in Canada (15) has assessed the direct medical costs of fibromyalgia syndrome to patients and to the general economy. The findings indicated that the annual direct medical cost of FMS to affected individuals was approximately $2,275.00. When this was multiplied by the 2 percent documented prevalence of FMS in the general population (8,9), the medical cost of this disorder to the U.S. economy has been estimated to be $12-15 billion annually and the Canadian cost appears to be comparable on a per capita basis. These costs can be divided approximately equally into three categories: (14); hospitalization costs, outpatient care costs, and medication administration costs. Hospitalization for the management of FMS pain finds little justification (16-19). A common reason for hospital admission is to exclude alternate diagnoses, but this can be accomplished more efficiently as an outpatient. It is also important that the physician does not assume that a variety of symptoms are due to FMS when other important inter-current medical conditions may just as likely intervene in these patients as in any other. With better education of physicians and increased awareness of FMS, consideration of this diagnosis early in the patient's course and effective outpatient care may lessen hospitalization care and its associated costs.

D. Taxonomy of FMS

The FMS is properly classified as one of a large group of *soft-tissue pain syndromes*. Some authors and many clinicians have improperly referred to this category of disorders generically as "myofascial pain disorders" but that confuses the issue with regard to a distinct disorder called "myofascial pain syndrome." Another taxonomic heading of past years was "non-articular rheumatism" but that term is too dated to be currently acceptable. The large group of soft tissue pain syndromes are characterized by pain which emanates from periarticular structures located outside of the joint capsule and periosteum. They differ from arthritic disorders in that the synovial joints are not directly involved. The anatomic structures which appear to be symptomatic can include ligaments, tendons, fascia, bursae, and muscles. All of these soft tissue structures are

known to facilitate mechanical functions of the diarthrodial joints. Any of these structures can become painful and dysfunctional alone or in association with distinct inflammatory, autoimmune, arthritic, or endocrine disorders. The resultant physical dysfunction and compromise in quality of life can be as severe as that associated with any of the arthritic diseases, so these soft tissue pain syndromes are not benign.

The following Table 1 shows a contemporary taxonomy of soft tissue pain syndromes.

SOFT-TISSUE PAIN SYNDROMES

The main subheadings divide the syndromes into localized, regionalized, and generalized categories. Most of the "localized" conditions are believed to result from repetitive mechanical injury to inadequately conditioned tissues. They are often named anatomically and are disclosed by a typical history plus the exquisite tenderness elicited by digital palpation of the affected structures.

The syndromes with a regional distribution tend to result from "overuse" or other injury. Even though they may involve more than one type of body structure, they are still limited in anatomic scope to a region or body quadrant. The myofascial pain syndrome [MPS] is characterized by "trigger points" [TrPs, contrasted with the different phenomenon and term "tender points," TePs, of FMS] and has traditionally been managed by physiatrists or neurologists. The masticatory myofascial pain syndrome [MMPS] involves the temporomandibular

TABLE 1. Classification of Soft Tissues Pain [STP] Syndromes

Localized	Regionalized	Generalized
Entrapment syndrome [e.g., carpal tunnel syndrome]	Myofascial pain syndrome [MPS]	Fibromyalgia syndrome [FMS]
Tenosynovitis [e.g., biceps tendinitis]]	Masticatory myofascial pain syndrome [TMD]	Chronic fatigue syndrome [CFS]
Bursitis [e.g., trochanteric bursitis]	Chronic regional pain syndrome [CRPS, RSD]	Polymyalgia rheumatica [PMR]
Enthesopathies [e.g., tennis elbow]	Referred visceral pain [e.g., left shoulder pain due to angina]	Hypermobility syndrome [HMS]

Adapted from: Russell IJ: J Musculoske Pain 1(1):1-7, 1993.

joint and/or TrPs in the muscles of mastication which are typically treated by dentists. Several types of visceral pain can be referred to a musculoskeletal structure [e.g., angina felt in the shoulder or jaw], and the recently renamed chronic regional pain syndrome [CRPS, formerly, reflex sympathetic dystrophy] would be classified in this category.

The "generalized" category implies a systemic process which affects the musculoskeletal system in a more global manner. The chronic fatigue syndrome [CFS] has been characterized by persistent idiopathic fatigue and a number of other constitutional symptoms. It initially presented in epidemics but more recent applications of that diagnosis have emphasized sporadic cases and the current criteria no longer exclude FMS. An overlap between FMS and CFS has led to speculation that they are identical but there are important historical and clinical differences which suggest that they are separate family members of an overlapping soft tissue pain spectrum. People with FMS report chronic widespread pain and are characterized by tenderness to palpation at many of the same anatomic sites involved in some of the localized pain syndromes.

DIAGNOSTIC PROTOCOL

A. Canadian Clinical Working Case Definition of FMS

The two compulsory pain criteria [adopted from the American College of Rheumatology 1990 Criteria (1)] are merged with Additional Clinical Symptoms & Signs to expand the classification of FMS into a Clinical Working Case Definition of FMS.
1. *Compulsory HISTORY of widespread pain.* Pain is considered widespread when all of the following are present for at least three months: • pain in both sides of the body • pain above and below the waist [including low back pain] • axial skeletal pain [cervical spine, anterior chest, thoracic spine or low back]. Shoulder and buttock involvement counts for either side of the body. "Low back" is lower segment.
2. *Compulsory PAIN ON PALPATION at 11 or more of the 18 defined tender point sites.* • *Occiput [2]*–at the suboccipital muscle insertions [see Figure 1] • *Low cervical [2]*–at the anterior aspects of the intertransverse spaces [the spaces between the transverse processes] at C5-C7 • *Trapezius [2]*–at the midpoint of the upper border • *Supraspinatus [2]*–at origins, above the scapular spine near its medial border • *Second rib [2]*–just lateral to the second costochondral junctions, on the upper rib surfaces • *Lateral epicondyle [2]*–2 cm distal to the epicondyles [in the brachioradialis muscle] • *Gluteal [2]*–in upper outer quadrants of buttocks in the anterior fold of muscle • *Greater trochanter [2]*–posterior to the trochanteric prominence • *Knee [2]*–at medial fat pad proximal to the joint line
3. *Additional clinical symptoms & signs.* In addition to the compulsory pain and tenderness required for research classification of FMS, many additional clinical symptoms and signs can contribute importantly to the patients' burden of illness. Two or more of these features are present in most FMS patients by the time they seek medical attention. On the other hand, it is uncommon for any individual FMS patient to have all of the associated symptoms or signs. As a result, the clinical presentation of FMS may vary somewhat, and the patterns of involvement may eventually lead to the recognition of FMS clinical subgroups.

These additional clinical symptoms and signs are not required for the research classification of FMS but they are still clinically important. For these reasons, the following clinical symptoms and signs are itemized and described in an attempt to expand the compulsory pain criteria into a proposed Clinical Case Definition of FMS [see Appendix 2, p. 79].

- *Neurological manifestations:* Neurological difficulties are often present such as hypertonic and hypotonic muscles; musculoskeletal asymmetry and dysfunction involving muscles, ligaments and joints; atypical patterns of numbness and tingling; abnormal muscle twitch response, muscle cramps, muscle weakness, and fasciculations. Headaches, temporomandibular joint disorder, generalized weakness, perceptual disturbances, spatial instability, and sensory overload phenomena often occur.
- *Neurocognitive manifestations:* Neurocognitive difficulties usually are present. These include impaired concentration and short-term memory consolidation, impaired speed of performance, inability to multi-task, easy distractibility, and/or cognitive overload.
- *Fatigue:* There is persistent and reactive fatigue accompanied by reduced physical and mental stamina, which often interferes with the patient's ability to exercise.
- *Sleep dysfunction:* Most FMS patients experience unrefreshing sleep. This is usually accompanied by sleep disturbances including insomnia, frequent nocturnal awakening, nocturnal myoclonus, and/or restless leg syndrome.
- *Autonomic and/or neuroendocrine manifestations:* These manifestations include cardiac arrhythmias, neurally mediated hypotension, vertigo, vasomotor instability, sicca syndrome, temperature instability, heat/cold intolerance, respiratory disturbances, intestinal and bladder motility disturbances with or without irritable bowel or bladder dysfunction, dysmenorrhea, loss of adaptability and tolerance for stress, emotional flattening, lability, and/or reactive depression.
- *Stiffness:* Generalized or even regional stiffness that is most severe upon awakening and typically lasts for hours as occurs with active rheumatoid arthritis. It can return during periods of inactivity during the day.

FIGURE 1. Location of Fibromyalgia Syndrome Tender Points [TrPs]

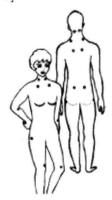

B. Application Notes

1. *Digital Palpation*

   The palpation examination should be performed with an approximate force of 4 kg/1.4 cm² [pressure required to partially blanch the blood from under the thumbnail]. This force can be standardized by pressing thumb on a weight scale. For a tender point to be considered "positive," the subject must state that the palpation was painful. "Tender" is not to be considered "painful."

2. *Validity*

   The two compulsory pain criteria were validated as classification criteria applicable to groups of subjects for the purpose of research study. In that setting, they yielded 88.4 percent sensitivity and 81.1 percent specificity. They have not yet been validated for clinical diagnosis of symptomatic individuals in a medical care setting.

3. *Focus of the Clinical Working Case Definition*

   In a clinical setting, the physician must appreciate the spectrum of FMS and the range of distress it can cause. Thus, in addition to identifying FMS using the two compulsory pain features, the clinician should assess the patient for other symptoms and signs that typically embody FMS in order to establish the patient's total illness burden and direct appropriate treatment in a timely fashion. The following hour-glass diagram indicates the steps to be followed by first narrowing the compulsory pain features to establish the classification of FMS and then expanding the spectrum of the additional symptoms and signs to determine the patient's total illness burden.

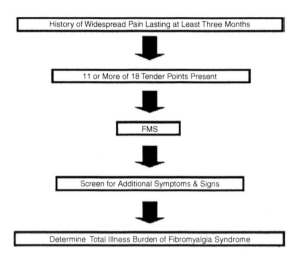

C. General Considerations in Applying the Clinical Case Definition to an Individual Patient

1. *Assess Patient's Total Illness*
   The clinical status of FMS is arrived at by consideration of the total burden of illness on the patient's life. This requires an assessment of all of the patient's symptoms, as well as a working knowledge of the demands associated with the patient's lifestyle, occupation, etc.

2. *Seek Evidence for Coherence of Symptoms*
   The patient's symptoms should fit a pattern that is identifiable as FMS.

3. *Identify Co-Existent Secondary Symptoms and Aggravators*
   It is important to distinguish the direct symptoms and signs of FMS from the sequelae of a chronic illness, daily chronic pain, loss of productivity, and non-supportive family members or acquaintances.

4. *Quantify the Severity of the Major Symptoms, and Their Impact on Lifestyle*
   An assessment of the severity of each major symptom, quantified on a symptom hierarchy/severity scale, and their impact on the patient's life is important in developing a treatment program and in assessing disability and prognosis. Compare the symptoms severity and impact to the patient's premorbid state of health and activity level.

D. Discussion of Major Features of FMS: Clinical Observations

It is suggested that the clinician use the compulsory pain and tenderness criteria to make a positive classification of FMS. Then, the clinician can ascertain the presence or absence of the additional symptoms and signs to apply this more comprehensive Clinical Working Case Definition [diagnosis] of FMS to a given individual. The defining symptom of FMS remains widespread chronic pain that lasts at least three months. The second compulsory criterion of a positive tender point examination would still apply to only a proportion of those meeting the first compulsory criterion. The additional clinical symptoms and signs [including neurological manifestations, fastigue, disturbed sleep, cognitive dysfunction, autonomic/neuroendocrine manifestations, and stiffness] provide relevant detail to the composite picture of the affected individual and more fully reflect the actual pathogenesis underlying his/her clinical illness. This more complete recognition of the scope of the illness provides the clinician with an expanded basis for understanding the patient and individualizing available therapy. Early diagnosis is important and may lessen the overall impact of FMS.

1. *Pain and Neurological Manifestations*

   a. *Characteristics of FMS Pain*
      Patients may describe their pain as any combination of burning, searing, tingling, shooting, stabbing, deep aching, sharp, and/or feeling bruised all over. Characteristics of FMS pain include:

- *Allodynia* is a reduction in pain threshold resulting in pain from a stimulus that normally would not be painful [hyper-excitability and super susceptibility], e.g., painful tender points
- *Hyperalgesia* is an abnormally high sensitivity to pain. Upon application of a stimulus that is ordinarily painful, the person perceives a greater intensity of pain than that stimulus would be expected to produce [super reactivity].
- *Persistent pain:* After a painful stimulus, pain persists for a longer duration than normal [super duration of response].
- *Pronounced summation effects and after-reaction* to repetitive stimuli.
- *Hyperpathia in skin:* When a point of a pin is drawn across the skin, it is felt more sharply over affected dermatomes.
- *Tenderness on examination:* It is also important to recognize that the widespread pain, and painful tenderness to palpation on physical examination, are two separate and independent entities that often change independently. The designated eighteen tender points of FMS were chosen because they were the most diagnostically discriminatory in the studies leading up to the development of ACR criteria. These criteria state that a tender point has a lowered pain threshold if it is perceived as painful when an approximate force of 4 kg/1.4 cm^2 [approximate area used by the palpating thumb] is applied to it. This is the force necessary to partially blanch the blood from under the nail plate of the palpating thumb. Many FMS patients have pain at a much lighter pressure than this. Elicited tender point pain does not shoot or radiate to a distant site, nor is it necessary that the examiner feel taut bands or nodules within the underlying muscle, although they are sometimes felt.

The periosteum [outer layer of bone], ligaments, tendons, fascia [the connective tissue that surrounds the muscle], and muscles are sensitive to pain (20). The tender points in FMS are primarily where ligaments, tendons and muscles attach to the bone. Ligaments are flexible but cannot stretch very far. A common cause of chronic muscle spasm and pain is ligament laxity. Loose ligaments cannot stabilize the joint and allow the joint to move beyond its normal range of motion producing painful sensations and numbness and tingling. Injuries to ligaments, such as whiplash injuries or back strain, can over-stretch, tear and/or fray the cable-like structure of ligaments (21). Unlike muscles, ligaments have a poor blood supply, particularly at the point where they attach to the bone. Thus ligaments often do not heal completely and can remain in a "stretched-out" position. When weakened ligaments or tendons are stretched or the joints are moved too much, sensory nerves can become irritated or compressed, causing local and/or referred pain (21). The abnormal joint movement creates many protective actions by adjacent tissues. Muscles will contract and become taut and shortened in an attempt to pull the joint back to its correct position, or to stabilize it and protect it from further damage.

b. *Other Features of FMS Pain*

- *Widespread pain:* Pain is considered widespread when it is felt globally; that is, bilaterally, and above and below the waist. Widespread pain may originate from a soft tissue injury such as whiplash, which initiates a local or regional myofascial pain syndrome, with regional tender and/or trigger points. Over a course of months, the globalization of body pain with multiple tender points, meeting the criteria of FMS, suggest that there are changes and abnormalities in the interaction between the peripheral nervous system and the CNS pain processing.
- *Non-anatomical distribution:* The pain is usually generalized and in "non-anatomical" distributions or regional, in that it does not follow any definite structural or nerve root distributions. It often includes a generalized myalgia, not necessarily confined to the eigh-

teen classical tender points used in physical examination. Usually it is perceived as originating in the muscles or deep in bones, and the character of the pain varies widely even in an individual patient. The pain also shifts, occurring in unexpected places at unexpected times, and can change day to day, or even hour to hour.

- *There is a delay in onset* after precipitating injury or prodromal event.
- *Pain can be felt in regions of perceived sensory deficit.*
- *Diffuse arthralgia* [pain in joints] occurs without joint swelling or redness, the lack of which differentiates FMS arthralgia from frank arthritis. This is an important distinction, since studies show that the body pain of FMS can be as severe as joint pain in RA (22,17).
- *Shortness of breath, and chest pain* is often experienced, which is reminiscent of, but usually distinguishable from angina. Commonly the chest pain of FMS is referred to as "atypical chest pain."
- *Low back pain* is common and is sometimes accompanied by pain that shoots down the leg, simulating sciatica. In that case, there may be concomitant piriformis muscle myofascial pain with compression of the sciatic nerve.
- *Leg cramps:* Approximately 40 percent of FMS patients reported leg cramps in comparison to 2 percent of controls (23,24).
- *Generalized stiffness,* which is worse upon awakening, commonly occurs in FMS. In studies of 78 patients and 973 patients, the reported incidence of morning stiffness lasting more than fifteen minutes was 79 percent (25). and 83 percent (26).
- *Chronic headache* is a common problem and can be very severe. Chronic daily headache typically involve excessive tension of cervical muscles and include muscle contraction [tension] headaches associated with neck and shoulder girdle pain but uncommonly true migraine. In studies of 78 and 973 patients, the reported incidence of

chronic headaches was 58 percent (25) and 49 percent (26), respectively.

c. *Other Neurological Manifestations*

- *Hypersensitivity to sense of vibration*
- *Positive Romberg test*
- *Abnormal tandem gait*
- *Abnormal serial seven subtraction testing is common.* Distraction tends to aggravation this difficulty, e.g., performance of tandem gait and serial sevens at the same time. This phenomenon may be most evident even when the baseline serial sevens test and tandem gait are both normal when done individually.
- *Abnormal twitch response* when there is associated MPS [see Appendix 4, p. 85].
- *Muscle weakness and fasciculations, and/or general weakness*
- *Atypical patterns of numbness and tingling* [dysesthesia] are often experienced in the hands or feet and sometimes are accompanied by a sense of swelling. Because of these symptoms, many patients undergo carpal tunnel syndrome [CTS] release surgery, only to experience no change in the tingling or pain. Therefore, FMS patients should not have carpal tunnel release surgery unless objective clinical manifestations of CTS are present [thenar wasting or weakness of opponens strength] and median nerve injury is confirmed by EMG/NCV studies. Subjective numbness was reported by 64 percent of the patients in one study (25).
- *Perceptual disturbances abound:* Lack of ability to make figure/ground distinctions, loss of depth perception or inability to focus vision and attention may be experienced. Affected individuals may lose portions of the visual field or can only make sense of a small portion of it at one time.
- *Temporal instability:* There are dimensional disturbances of timing, which affect the ability to sequence actions and perceptions.
- *Spatial instability* comes in many varieties, with gait tracking problems,

loss of cognitive mapping and inaccurate body boundaries–e.g., one bumps into the side of the doorway on trying to go through it and/or walks off the sidewalk. There may be an inability to automatically "attune" to the environment, as in accommodating footfall to irregular ground while walking and temporary loss of basic habituated motor programs such as walking, brushing one's teeth, making the bed and/or dialing a telephone.

- *Overload phenomena* affect sensory modalities where the patient may be hypersensitive to light, sound, noise, speed, odors, and mixed sensory modalities. Motor overload is exemplified by patients becoming clumsy as they fatigue, and stagger and stumble as they try to walk, unable to hold to a straight line, as well as showing generalized and local weakness. All of these cognitive, motor and perceptual disturbances may be associated with dizziness, numbness, tinnitus, nausea or shooting pain. There can be emotional overload from extraneous emotional fields such as excessive busyness, anger, and depression that unduly disturb the patient. These overload phenomena may precipitate a "crash." They can present in symptom clusters, which are usually quite unique to the patient.

- *Myelopathy from cervical cord compression* can cause abnormal long tract signs and local dysfunction at the cervical roots involved. This is not considered to be a cause of FMS but structural spinal abnormalities, including cervical cord compression, can mimic FMS. [See discussion of the work of Heffez et al. (27) in the pathogenesis discussion section, M. CNS Imaging, Functional Imaging Studies.] Therefore, a thorough neurological examination should be done, especially looking at the following (28):

  - *Motor system:* Check strength, bulk, tone, and the presence of tremor.
  - *Sensory system:* Check for sharp-dull pain discrimination, posterior column sensations including joint position and vibration sense with Romberg testing
  - *Cerebellar function:* Check drift, nystagmus, tandem gait, finger to nose, heel on shin, and rapid alternating motion.
  - *Cranial nerves:* Standard testing protocol when indicated by symptoms or signs.
  - *Reflexes:* Particularly look for long tract signs, clonus, Babinski's sign, Hoffman's sign, and radial periosteal, and flexor digitorum profundus reflexes. These reflex assessments should also be accomplished during neck flexion and extension. If abnormalities are accentuated, this suggests underlying long tracts of the cervical cord.
  - *Cognitive:* Conduct a mini-mental status assessment when symptoms or signs indicate.

Even after the criteria for FMS are met, abnormalities on neurological examination should prompt the same consideration of neurological imaging of the central nervous system or the spine as would be performed if FMS were not present. The imaging protocol may include magnetic resonance imaging [MRI] of the foramen magnum and cervical spine. [See Appendix 10 for instructions for a MRI.] Early diagnosis and treatment of spinal stenosis is important, because the degree of success from surgical or non-surgical treatment is inversely proportional to the duration of symptoms. It is usually not useful to perform MRIs on patients with normal neurological examinations.

2. *Neurocognitive Dysfunction*
Some FMS patients will suffer from a subset of symptoms that can be triggered as a cluster. Apart from the subset of patients with cervical myelopathy, neurocognitive symptoms are generally more severe in patients who also meet the diagnostic criteria for myalgic encephalomyelitis/chronic fatigue syndrome [ME/CFS]. These symptoms are more characteristically variable

than constant since they usually reflect cognitive fatigue rather than fixed impairment. Especially common are cognitive "fog" or simple confusion, trouble with linguistic performance, dyslexia that is exhibited only when the patient is fatigued, trouble with writing, reading, mathematics, word retrieval and speaking, short-term memory consolidation, as well as ease of interference with multi-tasking and background disturbances. It is easy for patients to lose track of things and/or many things are forgotten: names, numbers, sentences, conversations, appointments, their intentions and plans, where things are in the house, where they left the car or if they brought the car, where they are and where they are going. This memory dysfunction primarily affects short-term memory. There can also be cognitive overload including information overload, inability to multi-task, and trouble making decisions, which can lead to a "crash."

3. *Fatigue*

Patients exhibit general fatigue that is generally worse in the morning and they often awaken feeling more exhausted than when they went to bed. The fatigue is often associated with diffuse pain and stiffness. In summary reports of 78 and 973 FMS patients, the reported incidence of fatigue was 87 percent (25) and 75 percent (26), respectively. Fatigue may be generated by many different mechanisms. The following classification may be helpful in assessing fatigue (29).

a. *Structural Fatigue*

Failure of the supportive structure to withstand further pressure/load is caused by abnormalities of the skeleton, usually in the joints or discs. Fatigue of this type is influenced by the duration of weight bearing. It can be associated with pain and, in the case of the spine, the patient may have to sit down or lie down in order to get relief; however, sleep is not usually required but recovery is prolonged. This type of fatigue is common in FMS.

b. *Muscular Fatigue*

Muscular fatigue is associated with muscle dysfunction, of paretic or spastic type. The former is associated with decreased muscle bulk/tone while the latter by increased muscle bulk/tone. Muscular fatigue is brought on by movement and relieved by stopping the motion, but recovery is often moderately long. Unlike structural fatigue, movement is necessary to generate pain. Muscular fatigue is commonly seen in FMS and cervical stenosis.

c. *Arousal Fatigue*

Arousal fatigue results from an inadequate quantity or quality of sleep and can also be caused by some pharmaceuticals. This type of fatigue requires sleep for recovery. Most FMS patients do not get enough restorative slow wave sleep so this is a typical cause fatigue in FMS. The recovery period varies depending on the cause or the extent of the sleep debt.

d. *Motivational Fatigue*

The patient lacks the emotional drive to undertake activity. Physical performance is not impaired by motivational fatigue. Neither sleep nor rest makes a difference. This type of fatigue is usually associated with depression which is present in about 30 percent of FMS patients.

e. *Oxygenation Fatigue*

Oxygenation fatigue results from the inability of the body to deliver enough oxygen to the tissues. It has been proposed that this form of fatigue is caused by inadequacy of oxygen carrying capacity [hemoglobinopathy or anemia], poor circulation [heart failure, local ischemia caused by arterial blockage or venous stasis], or failure of oxygen transfer [respiratory disease or failure]. Fatigue of this type is often associated with increased breathing/heart rate and usually is relieved by simply stopping the activity without need to change posture. Recovery is usually rapid when the cause is corrected. Patients with FMS who have severe chest wall pain can so severely limit chest wall motion as to develop alveolar hypoventilation. They become hypoxic despite normal cardiorespiratory anatomy. The solution is to educate and control the chest wall pain.

f. *Metabolic Fatigue*

Metabolic abnormalities of the tissue whereby the cells are unable to transform energy substrates into useful functions can result in metabolic fatigue. This fatigue occurs as a result of inadequate hormonal physiology, such as hypothyroidism and adrenal insufficiency, or intrinsic metabolic abnormalities such as mitochondrial dysfunction. The fatigue is generalized and is not correctable unless the metabolic abnormality is corrected.

In FMS, the fatigue would seem to be unexpected or inappropriate, and there is often a delayed reactivity following physical exertion, with the onset the next day or even later. Such reactive or delayed fatigue may be associated with increased pain or impaired cognitive function. Thus, fatigue is correlated with other symptoms, often in a sequence that is unique to each patient. Patients who develop FMS often lose the natural antidepressant effect of exercise, feeling worse after exercise rather than better. After relatively normal physical or intellectual exertion, a patient may take an inordinate amount of time to regain the pre-exertion level of function and competence. This problem may resolve with use of pyridostigmine prior to aerobic exercise because it reverses the blockade of growth hormone by somatostatin in FMS [see p. 39].

4. *Sleep Dysfunction*

Most patients experience sleep and other diurnal rhythm disturbances that may include early, middle or late insomnia, hypersomnia, abnormal diurnal variation of energy levels, including reversed or chaotic irregularly irregular diurnal rest and sleep rhythms. Loss of the deeper phases of sleep [not spending enough time in stages three and four sleep] is especially characteristic, with frequent awakenings, and loss of restorative feelings on awakening. It may be accompanied by restless leg syndrome and periodic limb movement disorder. In studies of 78 and 973 patients, the reported incidence of poor sleep was 82 percent (25) and 60 percent (26), respectively. Nocturnal myoclonus has been reported in over 50 percent of FMS patients in one study (30). Restless leg syndrome has been reported in approximately 30 percent of FMS patients compared to 2 percent of controls (24). Treatable sleep disorders such as upper airway resistance syndrome, obstructive and central sleep apnea should considered and tested for when indicated.

A research study by Moldofsky et al. (6) found that healthy normal controls [HNC], who were deprived of stage 4 sleep by means of a variety of auditory stimuli, may exhibit painful tender points upon palpation. This finding suggests that sleep disturbance is important in the genesis of tender points. Thus, it is important to distinguish between patients who simply need to adjust their schedule to get adequate sleep from those who have an inability to receive adequate restorative sleep.

5. *Autonomic and/or Neuroendocrine Dysfunctions*

a. *Autonomic Dysfunctions*

There is general loss of internal homeostasis and adaptation involving dysfunction of the autonomic system. There can be interaction between pain and autonomic phenomena.

• *Dizziness, neurally mediated hypotension [NMH], and vertigo:* The most common type of dizziness in fibromyalgia is a transient sense of imbalance that may be accompanied by a sense of lightheadedness. This transient dizziness is often brought on or associated with neck extension or quick rotation. The episodes are transient and rarely cause patients to fall. They are of short duration if the patient is still. This may be seen in patients who also have cervical disc disease. It may be caused by the transient contact of the cord against the bony spinal canal, causing transient distortion of proprioception. Once the patient becomes still, the cord floats away and the signals become reestablished with resolution of symptoms. In a study (31) of NMH in FMS patients, all 18 of 20 patients who were able to tolerate a 70 degree tilt for 10 minutes on a tilt table, had worsening of widespread pain whereas the controls remained asymptomatic. NMH can include symptoms of light-headedness, while rising from a sitting position or standing, cognitive difficulties, blurred vision, pallor, severe fatigue, tremulousness, and unexplained syncope. The less common but more troublesome form is vertigo in which the patient complains of the room spinning and often is accompanied by nystagmus, nausea and/or vomiting and is often incapacitating for hours to days. Sometimes vertigo is associated with tinnitus, suggestive of eighth nerve or vestibular malfunction. There is often some impaired hearing acuity, which is seen more often in patients who have had head trauma.

- *Loss of thermostatic and vasomotor stability* may be experienced as altered body temperature [usually subnormal] or hot and cold feelings, vasomotor instability, sometimes in unusual distribution, e.g., the right side may feel hot while the left feels cold, or there may be localized feelings of heat and flushing. Vasoconstriction generally differentiates neuropathic pain from inflammatory pain.

  With neuropathic pain, affected parts of the body are perceptibly colder, and retained catabolites from ischemia may exacerbate the pain. There may be increased sudomotor activity, with excessive sweating following painful movements. The pilomotor reflex is often hyperactive and visible in affected dermatomes ["goose-bumps"]. A stimulus such as chilling, which excites the pilomotor response, can precipitate pain; and vice versa. Pressure upon a tender motor point tends to provoke the pilomotor and sudomotor reflexes. The pilomotor reflex can often be augmented by pressing upon a tender point, especially the upper trapezius.

- *Neurogenic or trophic edema:* Patients with FMS often have swelling of the hands and feet or generalized swelling that may result from inactivity. Increased tone in lymphatic vessel smooth muscle and increased permeability in blood vessels can lead to local subcutaneous tissue edema. It has been reported that skin over a muscle exhibiting concomitant myofascial pain syndrome can exhibit the peau d'orange effect [orange peel skin] or a positive "matchstick" test. Trophic edema is non-pitting to digital pressure but when a blunt instrument is used, such as the end of a wooden matchstick, the indentation produced is clear-cut and persists for minutes and may be surrounded by "histaminic flare" reaction and occasionally wheals. Other tropic changes may occur in the skin and nails and there may be dermatomal loss of hair.

- *Sicca syndrome:* Patients may have chronic dry eyes and mouth. These sicca symptoms are present in about 30 percent of FMS patients while 50-60 percent of Sjögren's syndrome patients have FMS. In either situation, the contributions of anticholinergic drugs to the sicca symptoms must be considered.

- *Respiratory and cardiac irregularities:* Patients may experience breathing dysregulation, heart rate regulation abnormalities, and/or cardiac arrhythmias. Chest wall pain may be an important contributor to alveolar hypoventilation.

- *Intestinal irregularities and bladder dysfunction:* Intestinal irregularities and hypersensitivity to pain, i.e.,–irritable bowel syndrome [IBS]–diarrhea, constipation, alternating diarrhea and constipation, abdominal cramps and bloating are common symptoms in FMS. The IBS has been reported in 40 percent or more of FMS patients in comparison to approximately 15 percent or healthy controls (32). The IBS may be associated with severe L5-S1 disc disease or spinal stenosis in some patients. Bladder dysfunction is often associated with allodynia and pain sensitivity. Urinary frequency, dysuria, and nocturia, are also common.

b. *Neuroendocrine Dysfunctions*

- *Loss of adaptability:* There may be loss of adaptability and stress tolerance associated with dysfunction of the hypothalamic/pituitary/adrenal [HPA] axis (33).
- Marked weight gain is commonly seen. It has been suggested that hypothyroidism occurs approximately three to twelve times more often in FMS than in the general public (25) However, the most common causes of weight gain in FMS are probably similar to that of the general population, including a disproportion between dietary intake and calories burned by exercise.
- *Dysmenorrhea* is common.

6. *Other Associated Signs*

Musculoskeletal asymmetry and dysfunction involving muscles, ligaments and joints result in weakened, shortened tissues. Janda and Schmid (34-36) identified a number of muscular and postural changes associated with pain in a relevant and consistent relationship. In thorough and comprehensive examinations of the musculoskeletal system of approximately 2,000 FMS patients, Seibel (37) found that not only do virtually all FMS patients exhibit many of these muscular and postural changes, but he also identified numerous other changes and clinical signs associated with the musculoskeletal system. The following musculoskeletal imbalance patterns and other signs may be helpful in the clinical assessment of the FMS patient *but not necessarily unique to the FMS:*

a. *Muscle Shortening from Spasm*

Shortening of muscles from spasm results in muscle dysfunction. This fundamental feature may be due to spasm in the early phase of injury and referred to as the neuromuscular dysfunction phase [i.e., increased muscle tension due to non-voluntary motor nerve activity and seen on an electromyography as continuous

motor unit activity]. It can be due to contracture in the later stage of injury and referred to as the dystrophic phase [localized bands of spontaneous muscle shortening that are not due to continuous motor unit activity, and therefore no action potentials are revealed by electromyography]. Muscle shortening can often be palpated as ropy bands within muscles, which are sometimes fibrotic [contractures] in long standing conditions. The bands are seldom limited to individual muscles, but are present in muscle groups according to the pattern of neuropathy. The taut muscles appear weaker than normal. However, the muscles are dysfunctional due to their shortened state. Muscles must be examined and tight muscles must be stretched before exercising as rigorous exercise will cause further shortening and dysfunction of the shortened muscles, and produce pain. [See Treatment Protocol, D. Self-Powered FMS Exercise Programs.]

- *Limitation of joint range* may result from shortening of muscles, which can be caused by injured, weakened, and/or lax ligaments and/or tendons.
- *Enthesopathy:* Tendinous attachments to bone are often thickened in chronic cases of FMS or the diagnosis is confused with an inflammatory enthesopathic condition such as ankylosing spondylitis, Reiter's syndrome, or the musculoskeletal manifestations of inflammatory bowel disease.

b. *Head and Neck Are Too Far Forward*

A number of musculoskeletal changes are associated with this posture:

- There is shortening of the sub-occipital extensors, which causes extension of the occipital atlantal joints. This extension may cause restriction or impingement of the vertebral arteries and dural tube, which may contribute to some of the CNS symptoms in FMS.
- The mid-cervical facet joints are forward-bending.
- There is tightening of the long occipital extensors, such as the splenius capitis,

which in turn may trap and compress the lesser and greater occipital nerves, and give rise to headaches in the distribution of these nerves.

- There is an imbalance between the anterior cervical muscles, including the supra and infra hyoids, and the posterior cervical extensor.
- The posterior-lateral muscle bulk is smaller than the anterior-lateral muscle bulk [the posterior-lateral bulk should be 1.5 times that of the anterior-lateral]. This muscular bulk imbalance stretches the muscles and their attachments along the nuchal ridge, which is also a common source of headaches. A number of tight bands in the posterior cervical muscles, especially the splenius capitis, often can be found upon palpation.
- The nuchal ligament from the base of the skull to the spinous process of C6 can be found on palpation to feel like a "bow string" and thus, does not support the weight of the head and neck.
- There is a variable degree of loss of range of motion of the cervical spine.
- The sternocleidomastoids are short and tight and often contain trigger points, which refer to the head and can give signs and symptoms of migraine headaches (38).
- The scalenes are short and tight. Their usual function as cervical flexors is lost due to their origins along the lateral cervical spine now being anterior to their insertions to the first and second ribs. When the scalenes are short and tight, they may pull the first rib up to the clavicle. Dr. Seibel, in his assessment of approximately 2,000 patients, found the first rib is more often, but not always, elevated on the right as the right first rib is higher than the left and the right clavicle is lower than the left. This can compress the passing nerves and blood vessels, resulting in signs and symptoms of Thoracic Outlet Syndrome. The scalenes with their attachments to the first and second ribs also function as accessory muscles in respiration.

- There is an imbalance between the actions of the sternocleidomastoid, the levator scapulae and the trapezius.
- There are anterior and posterior restrictions of the first rib articulations.
- The muscular imbalance leads to abnormal muscle firing.
- The imbalance of the anterior and posterior cervical muscles can eventually result in degenerative joint disease from C4 through C7, and the T4 segment.
- The head and neck forward position can give rise to myofascial trigger points in related muscles in the neck, arms, shoulders and upper back, which results in pain and/or other symptoms in the classical referral patterns of such muscles.
- There may be supraclavicular swelling without adenopathy, which may be a possible sign of cord irritation (39).

c. *Postural and Muscular Imbalance Patterns and Signs of the Upper Body*

- The shoulders are elevated and adducted forward with tight levator scapulae, upper trapezeii, pectoralis major and minor, serratus anterior, and scalenii. The middle and lower trapezeii are stretched and inhibited. There is protraction and internal rotation of the shoulder girdle, involving the latissimus, subscapularis, pectoralis, and terres major. The altered angle of the glenoid fossa, the head of the humerus, which was kept in place by the supraspinatus, becomes unstable with the upper trapezius attempting to stabilize the glenohumeral joint. Due to these changes, no muscle now has the proper angle of pull to support the shoulder.
- The altered axis of the glenohumeral joint, and overstressed shoulder joint, in turn overstress the cervico-cranial junction, the C4/C5 segment, and the T4 segment.
- Taut muscles and abnormal joint movement lead to restriction of joint capsules, loss of proprioception, and reduced body strength.

- *A simple test for upper body strength*, as it pertains to both muscles and ligaments, will predict the patient's function in tasks using his/her upper body. Have the patient hold her/his arms abducted to 90 degrees at the shoulder and time how long s/he can hold this position. [Four minutes or longer is considered normal and requires 40 percent of normal upper body strength.]

d. *Lateral View Postural and Muscular Imbalance Patterns and Signs*

- From a lateral view there is an increased cervical lordosis, thoracic kyphosis and lumbar lordosis, with a forward pelvic tilt.
- The lateral center of posture reveals the head and shoulders to be anterior to the hips, knees, and ankles. The left shoulder is usually more anterior than the right.

e. *Posterior View Postural and Muscular Imbalance Patterns and Signs*

- From the posterior view, the iliac crest is usually superior and posterior on the same side that the shoulder is lower [more often, the left side], with positive Kemps and Trendelenburg's tests, indicative of sacral-iliac joint fixation.
- The left scapula is usually inferior to the right and both scapulae are protracted.

f. *Anterior View Postural and Muscular Imbalance Patterns and Signs*

- The left medial aspect of the clavicle is more often superior to the right and the right first rib is usually superior to the left.
- The left shoulder is more often inferior to the right and the left iliac crest is again usually superior to the right.
- There usually is subluxation of C1 (40) and T12 (41) to the same side as the elevated iliac crest and subluxation of C2 to the opposite direction.
- Poor diaphragmatic breathing, due to inhibited expansion of the lower rib cage, can be observed. There may be restriction of the upper chest breathing due to pectoral girdle muscle tension, which also causes adduction of the shoulders. The shallow breathing is accompanied by increased activity of the accessory respiratory muscles, with a tendency to muscle overload.

g. *Major Muscular Imbalance Patterns of the Lower Body*

- Usually there can be shortening of the quadriceps muscles resulting in decreased flexion of the knee and common complaints of knee pain, buckling and problems going up and down stairs, squatting, etc.
- The hip flexors, notably the iliopsoas and rectus femoris, are short and tight resulting in decreased extension of the hips. This decreased extension results in a forward pelvic tilt, hip flexion, and an increased lumbar lordosis to maintain an upright posture. This imbalance, in turn, over-stresses the lumbar spine segments, particularly the L5/S1 and its disc, the hips, and as a compensation, the thoracolumbar junction at T12/L1.
- There is an imbalance between the tight, short hip flexors and lumbar errector spinae, with weakened, inhibited gluteal and abdominal muscles. The hamstrings, triceps surae, and adductors are tight. The tightened hamstrings and adductors are often the cause of low back pain. It is possible to reproduce the patient's back pain by stretching these muscles, and treatment of these tight muscles can eliminate the patient's back pain.

h. *Functional Short Leg and Scoliosis*

- FMS patients frequently have a functional short leg caused by assimilation [upslip] on one side of the pelvis due to spasm and/or contracture of the iliopsoas, quadratus lumborum, latissimus dorsii and incompetence of the sacroiliac ligaments. Dr. Seibel observed that the functional short leg occurs more often, but not always, on the left side.

- There is often a compensatory scoliosis of the lumbar spine with the convexity towards the side of the functional short leg and scoliosis of the thoracic spine with convexity in the opposite direction.

i. *Overall Appearance*
In severe cases one may recognize an alteration in the shape of the patient's body, which is an expression of the generalized muscle imbalance and dysfunction.

- From the back view of the patient, there are layers of hyper- and hypotrophied muscles. Hypertrophied muscles include the hamstrings, T12/L1 area, upper trapezius, and deep neck extensors. Hypotrophied muscles include the gluteii, and spinal erectors at L4, L5, and S1 area.
- The front view mainly reveals an imbalance between the abdominal rectii, which are hypotrophied, and the abdominal obliques, which are hypertrophied.

Note: In the above section, the side of the body on which a particular sign usually occurs is based on the findings of the evaluation of approximately 2,000 patients (37). However, these signs may also occur on the opposite side of the body.

D. Clincal Evaluation of Fibromyalgia Syndrome

Assess the total illness burden of the patient, taking a thorough history, a physical examination, and ordering investigations as indicated to rule out other active disease processes.

1. *Patient History*
A thorough history, including a complete description of the patient's complaints as well as estimating their severity and their impact on the patient's ability to function, must be taken before attempting to classify the illness.
   a. *Presenting Complaint*
   - date and time of onset
   - trigger or prodromal event, including a careful description of trauma or other triggering event, particularly noting events that cause sudden excessive vertical load on the spine, or lateral loads such as impact from collisions and falls with head injuries.
   - symptoms at onset
   - progression of symptoms
   - duration of symptoms
   - hierarchy of severity and quality of current symptoms
   - identify aggravating/ameliorating environmental factors
   - distinguish primary symptoms from secondary symptoms and aggravators
   - quantify severity of total burden of symptoms and current level of physical function
   b. *Past History*
   The past history should include a comprehensive traumatic history and the patient's response to earlier trauma.
   c. *Systems Review*
   Many symptoms involve more than one system. Attention should be paid to:
   - *Musculoskeletal system* including myalgia and/or arthralgia.
   - *CNS* including fatigue with post-exertional exacerbation, neurocognitive complaints, and headaches
   - *Autonomic and endocrine systems:* There is a general loss of homeostasis and adaptability: loss of sleep rhythm, loss of thermostatic stability, heat/cold intolerance, vasomotor instability; perceptual disturbances, anxiety, marked weight change, emotional flattening, etc.
   - *Cardiorespiratory system* including delayed postural hypotension, postural orthostatic tachycardia, arrhythmias

- *GI* and *GU system* including arrhythmias–Irritable Bowel Syndrome [IBS]; bladder dysfunction
- *Psychological:* Estimate general emotional state.

2. *Physical Examination*
   a. *Functional State of Systems*
   Clinical estimation of the state of functioning and conditioning of the standard body systems should be ascertained.
   b. *Musculoskeletal System*
   During the tender point examination, the patient must have pain on palpation of designated tender point sites to meet the diagnosis of FMS. Special attention must be paid to the presence or absence of joint swelling, inflammation, range of motion, quality of movement, and patterns of muscle tension and muscle consistence. Check for scoliosis, functional short leg, and patterns of muscular and postural imbalance. Test upper body strength. Patients should also be assessed for the presence of myofascial trigger points.
   c. *CNS*
   A focused neurological assessment including a standard examination for pathological reflexes such as Hoffman's sign, Babinski's sign, clonus and hyperreflexia, as well as during neck flexion and extension as these maneuvers will accentuate any compression of the underlying long tracts of the cervical cord. Tandem walk, both forwards and backwards, and Romberg test should be evaluated. Regular re-evaluation for clear signs of neurological disease should be performed every six to twelve months.
   d. *Cardiorespiratory System*
   A clinical estimation of the state of conditioning should be ascertained. Measure supine and standing blood pressure, examine the peripheral pulses and circulatory adequacy. Arrhythmias and low or erratic blood pressure should be noted.
   e. *Autonomic* and *Neuroendocrine System*
   Check for signs of thyroid, adrenal and pituitary dysfunction, vasomotor instability, low body temperature, and sicca syndrome.

3. *Laboratory and Investigative Protocol*
   There is no specific laboratory test for fibromyalgia syndrome. However, it is important to screen for other conditions that may resemble it or complicate its management.
   a. *Routine Laboratory Tests*
   CBC, ESR, protein electrophoresis, CPK, CRP and TSH tests should be done.
   Further testing: In addition to the routine laboratory tests, additional tests should be chosen on an individual basis depending on the patient's case history, clinical evaluation, laboratory findings, and risk factors for co-morbid conditions. Many of these tests may be ordered after referral to a specialist. Clinicians should carefully evaluate the cost/benefit ratio of any investigative test for each patient and avoid unnecessary duplication of tests.
   b. *Further Laboratory Testing*
   If indicated, additional investigations may be done including tests for pituitary-adrenal axis function, and status of calcium metabolic indicators such as iPTH and 24-hour urine collections for calcium and phosphorus. If indicated, consider serum magnesium, blood glucose, serum electrolytes, Fe, B12 and folate levels, creatinine, DHEA sulfate, liver function, and routine urinalysis. *Cardiac assessment* such as ECG and Holter-monitoring, and *neurological tests* such as electromyography, and nerve conduction tests may be indicated. *Special risk factors and/or comorbid conditions* may indicate the need for one or more of the following tests: rheumatoid factor, antinuclear antibody, diurnal cortisol levels, 24 hour urine free cortisol and/or other appropriate thyroid and adrenal testing, total and free testosterone, estradiol, osteoarthritis, Western blot test for Lyme disease, chest x-ray, and TB skin test.

c. *Imaging*
  - *X-rays* of the cervical and lumbar spine, with flexion and extension views, are useful to determine mechanical problems including malalignments.
  - *Total body bone scan* may be useful to rule out inflammatory or destructive lesions in the skeletal systems.
  - *MRI and CT:* Patients with an appropriate history or positive neurological findings should have MRI or CT of the relevant part of the spine, such as imaging of the neck in extension.

d. *Tilt-Table Testing*
  If NMH is suspected, it should be confirmed by tilt-table testing prior to prescribing medication.

e. *Sleep Studies*
  Sleep studies should be ordered if a treatable sleep disorder is suspected. They can also be useful to establish presence of alpha-wave intrusion in non-REM sleep that is typical of FMS.

f. *sEMG and qEEG*
  These tests can be useful when indicated by neurologic symptoms or signs but are expensive and their costs are not covered by provincial health plans.

If the patient has any abnormalities in the screening blood tests such as high ESR, abnormal ANA, RA, etc., it is recommended that the patient be monitored closely for a number of months to allow time for the maturation of symptoms that may be due to another condition. They may eventually warrant referral to a rheumatologist.

Concurrent conditions: Assuming the clinical criteria are satisfied, the presence of other medical conditions generally does not exclude the diagnosis of FMS. Restless leg syndrome, irritable bowel/bladder syndrome, vasomotor instability, and sicca may have a temporal coherence to FMS and may actually be part of the syndrome.

Differential diagnosis: There are many medical conditions that can be similarly characterized by widespread pain, paresthesia, stiffness, and/or fatigue. These include [see also Appendix 5, p . 82]:
Systemic immune arthropathies: e.g., rheumatoid arthritis, systemic lupus erythematosus, psoriatic arthritis, ankylosing spondylitis, polymyositis and temporal arteritis/polymyalgia rheumatica.
Skeletal malignancies such as multiple myeloma, bony metastases
Neuromuscular disorders including multiple sclerosis, myasthenia gravis, polyneuropathy
Endocrine disturbances including primary and secondary hyperparathyroidism, renal osteodystrophy, osteomalacia, hypothyroidism, hypoadrenalism
It is important not to attribute symptoms of FMS to other illnesses or visa versa, since it may lead to unnecessary and sometimes potentially toxic medications being prescribed.

Patients who meet the criteria for FMS should be evaluated to see if they also meet the criteria for myalgic encephalomyelitis/chronic fatigue syndrome [ME/CFS], since many of the symptoms are similar. The myofascial pain syndrome involving regional muscles should also be considered.

E. Differences Between Fibromyalgia Syndrome and Myalgic Encephalomyelitis/Chronic Fatigue Syndrome [ME/CFS]

A syndrome may be delineated by means of a criterion that reflects a cutoff point on a continuum of symptoms and dysfunctions. Patients with FMS and ME/CFS can be clinically differentiated on the basis of symptom balance in what some investigators believe are a variation of the same or similar pathogenesis. With respect to symptoms, FMS is at the extreme of the chronic pain spectrum, with lesser degrees of fatigue and cognitive disturbance. ME/CFS is at the extreme end of the chronic fatigue spectrum but often involves significant cognitive dysfunction and pain as well. It has been proposed that there are three groups of patients: those with pure FMS, those with pure ME/CFS, and patients who meet the criteria for both syndromes (42). One study suggests approximately 75 percent of ME/CFS patients also meet the criteria for FMS (43), but there is a much lower rate of FMS patients who meet the criteria for ME/CFS. Some fibromyalgia syndrome patients can develop ME/CFS and visa versa.

Another important difference between FMS and ME/CFS is in the response to exercise. Patients with mild FMS may be better able to tolerate exercise whereas it aggravates the symptoms in ME/CFS and severely afflicted FMS patients, who need alternate forms of exercise and a gentler progression. Patients with ME/CFS can be distinguished from healthy controls and FMS patients by determining the ratio of normal 80 kilodalton [kDa] ribonuclease L [RNase L] to the low molecular weight 37 kDa RNase L found in ME/CFS patients (44), but not characteristic of FMS. [See also Appendix 5, p. 82.]

A clear diagnosis often has a considerable therapeutic benefit as it reduces uncertainty and orients therapy, both specific and nonspecific.

. . . Dr. Bruce Carruthers, Canada

TREATMENT PROTOCOL

A. General Considerations

Once a physician is satisfied that the diagnosis of FMS is accurate, treatment of the patient must be individualized. The physician must understand that the treatment will take time and require regular follow-up. The approach should be all encompassing, with therapies carefully thought through and tailored to the diversity and severity of symptoms, to reduce the overall impact of the burden of illness on the patient. The modalities of therapy can be supported in specific individuals using $N = 1$ trial techniques if indicated. The patient must be carefully monitored to determine the effectiveness of treatment. The physician has a pivotal role in empowering and supporting the well-being of the patient, who is immersed in a climate of confusion and uncertainty. The patient should be involved through education, lifeworld adjustments, and the judicial use of pharmacological and non-pharmacological interventions. [See Appendices 11-19, pp. 90-104.]

B. Goals and Therapeutic Principles/ Guidelines to Help Structure Self-Powered Lifeworld Adjustments and Therapy

1. *Therapeutic Goal*
   A major therapeutic goal is to empower patients to trust their own experiences and enhance their ability to recognize the consistency of some symptoms and the fluctuation and interaction of others, so they can achieve a lifeworld environment in which they can be as active as possible without aggravating their symptoms, and then gradually expand their activity boundaries.

2. *Symptom Severity and Hierarchy Profile*
   At the initial assessment and periodically [every 6 months or so], patients should be asked to quantify the severity of the prominent FMS symptoms of pain, fatigue, sleep disturbance, cognitive difficulties, and make a hierarchy profile of those symptoms. [See Appendix 6-9, pp. 83-88.] Patients should also indicate their level of functionality and note the causal relationship between therapies or events that relieve or aggravate symptoms.

3. *Therapeutic Principles/Guidelines*

   a. *State of Well-Being Principle*
      The state of well-being involves the process whereby essential variables of the *body's internal environment* are kept within acceptable limits [homeostasis]. All therapy is aimed at assisting the body in returning to the pre-illness state of well-being, which must be balanced with orderly change [homeorrhesis].

   b. *The Treating Physician Knows the Patient Best*
      As the treating physician is most involved in and responsible for the ongoing care and well-being of the patient, he/she should direct and coordinate treatment and rehabilitation efforts.

   c. *Rehabilitation Personnel Must Be Knowledgeable About FMS.*

d. *The Pathophysiology of FMS Must Be Respected and Reflected in the Program.*

- *The complexities and interactive nature of the varied dysfunctions of FMS are a physiological reality of the illness and must be accommodated.*
- *The symptoms and activity boundaries of FMS patients fluctuate on a day to day and even an hour to hour basis.* Patients in the early stages of FMS tend to have more normal activity boundaries, while those with severe or long-standing symptoms have more limited activity boundary dynamics.
- *Avoid exacerbating the patient's symptoms.* The limitations of FMS are set by the abnormal physiology. Avoid severe and prolonged exacerbation of symptoms by developing interventions that the individual patient can tolerate.

e. *The Philosophy of the Program Is of Utmost Importance and Must Be Conducive to Healing.*

- *The program must reflect the patient's total illness burden:* The patient's impairments, their interactions, and any aggravating or extenuating circumstances, must be assessed and reflected in the program.
- *Empower the patient:* The autonomy of the patient is vital to his/her physical and psychological health. Support and enhance the patient's sense of self-empowerment through respect and involvement. The patient is directly aware of many of her/his body processes and should be encouraged to recognize and heed symptoms that are signals or warning signs from the body to change or modify activities.
- *Develop an appropriate individualized program:* The patient should be involved with establishing a program that is appropriate for his/her state of health, impairments and fluctuating activity boundaries.
- *Engage the patient in establishing realistic goals:* It is essential that the patient be able to establish the level of complexity and pace of her/his activities, have a sense of control over his/her environment, and be able to incorporate rest periods as needed.
  - *Begin the program* at the patient's base level of activity to ensure the patient's success.
  - *Pace the program* so that it gradually increases to coincide with the patient's increasing level of ability. This positive progress will ensure that the patient's continued commitment and success.
  - *Develop a plan of alternative strategies* for times when the patient is feeling poorly or has flare-ups.
- Optimize the patient's ability to function within her/his lifeworld.
- *Have the patient explore ways to gently extend his/her activity boundaries.*
- *Keep directions simple, clear, and concise.*
- *Establish a healing environment by using the Principle of the Four 'S'es– keep it simple, serene, slow, and supportive.* It should maximize healing resources and minimize stress, pain, overload phenomena, and adverse environmental exposures.

C. Self-Powered Lifeworld Adjustments and Self-Help Therapies

Patients often feel confused as they face the uncertainties of the significant physical, psychosocial and economic impact of having FMS. Hendriksson's research (45) indicated the five main symptoms influencing daily performance are chronic pain and muscular fatigue [present 90 percent of daytime–50 percent to a pronounced degree], tiredness, disturbed sleep, cognitive dysfunction and decreased muscle endurance. Regardless of whether or not patients are able to work, it is essential that they make appropriate self-powered lifeworld adjustments that will help them maximize their coping skills and become as self-reliant as possible. Physicians can assist patients in developing *individualized management programs that respect patients' autonomy and help them adapt to their limitations.* Some patients may benefit from an assessment by an occupational therapist [OT] who is knowledgeable about the particular problems surrounding FMS. The OT can alert them to various self-help practices, and assist them in modifying their daily routines.

1. *Patient Education*

    a. *Information About FMS and Sources of Support*

    A meeting with the patient and their meaningful others should be held as soon as possible after the diagnosis is made. Education on self-powered management is important. It is helpful to establish resources to enrich support and care, such as the National ME/FM Action Network, Fibromyalgia Network, National Fibromyalgia Research Association, Oregon Fibromyalgia Foundation, Co-Cure, provincial and state organizations, local support groups, articles, videos, etc. Information on FMS and related subjects as well as links for numerous international web sites can be found on the National ME/FM Action Network website (*http://www.mefmaction.net*)

    b. *Early Warning Signals*

    Encourage awareness of early warning signals of excessive fatigue, pain, and/or cognitive dysfunctions such as sensory over-stimulation, and provide ways to prevent "crashes"[1] and/or get early treatment. Assist patients in recognizing the activities and environments in which they can cope without exacerbating symptoms and to pace themselves accordingly. Patients should explore ways of gradually extending those boundaries at their own pace.

    c. *Establish a Healing Environment–Principle of the Four 'S'es–Simple, Serene, Slow, and Supportive*

    Assist patients in creating a simple, serene, and supportive environment that fits their pace, maximizes healing resources, and minimizes stress, pain and fatigue. Special attention should be given to avoiding or minimizing physical, cognitive, and psychosocial overload, and adverse environmental factors.

    d. *Relaxation and Stress Reduction Techniques*

    Patients should be encouraged to reduce stress and overload situations and incorporate rest and relaxation periods into their day. [See Appendix 15 for various relaxation techniques.]

    e. *Keep the Body Warm*

    When cold or experiencing severe, acute pain, patients should be encouraged to sit in a hot bath for 20 to 30 minutes or have a hot shower, then lie down and wrap up in blankets to keep as warm as possible. A hot water bottle or heating pad can be helpful. [See Appendix 12.]

    f. *Practical Energy Conservation Information, Environmental Modifications, and Functional Devices*

    Encourage patients to structure tasks and improve their consistency by making reminder notes and organizers to simplify routines including those of personal grooming, household chores such as food preparation and laundry, shopping and gardening. Environmental modifications include an appropriate arrangement of furniture, lighting and heating. Ergonomic considerations will help stabilize posture and facilitate movement (46) [Appendix 14]. Self-help items that will assist patients in their daily living include items such as the use of stretch stocking to reduce neurally mediated hypotension, various kinds of jar openers, reach and grab extensions, canes, yellow sunglasses to reduce the glare of headlights in evening driving, and the use of a sheet of yellow plastic on paper work to reduce eye strain.

    g. *Avoid Known Environmental Aggravators*

    Encourage patients to avoid or minimize exposure to any environmental aggravators that they have found to worsen their condition. The following aggravators for some patients may be overlooked:

    - overexertion
    - change in sleep schedule
    - overhead reaching
    - prolonged muscular or mental activity
    - excessive stress
    - air travel–jet lag, exposure to recirculating stale air and viruses, vestibular

nerve stimulation and excessive vibration
- exposure to extremes in temperature
- loud music and noise
- caffeine
- aspartame
- alcohol
- nicotine
- allergen exposure
- chemical exposure
- glutamate in additives, e.g., MSG

Do not misuse a tolerable day!

...Dr. Robert Olin
Karolinska Institute, Sweden

2. *Self-Development*

a. *Know and Trust Their Inner Feelings, Values, Needs, Sensitivities, and Experiences.*
Some patients may find journaling or creative writing helpful to bring insight to their feelings and provide a sense of well-being. They should enhance their communication skills to calmly let their needs and abilities known.

b. *Set Personal Boundaries*
Encourage patients to accept themselves despite their limitations, tame perfectionism, and learn to say, "No."

c. *Gradually Extend Emotional, and Perceptual/Cognitive Boundaries*
Patients should set aside a regular time to do activities they enjoy such as reading, solitaire, crossword puzzles, etc. Creative endeavors such as music and painting are relaxing and may help improve brain function and mood. Encourage patients to explore different ways to gradually include activities that will extend their boundaries.

3. *Maximizing Sleep*

a. *Pace Daytime Activities Appropriately*
Encourage patients to pace daytime activities appropriately to conserve energy. One such plan involves use of a timer device which is first set for a given period of time when the affected individual begins the work day. When that period of time has expired, the person resets the same time and must rest for an equal period of time or at least change to a different activity. Upon conclusion of the next period of time, the person can return to the original task. In this manner, the day is manditorially divided into segments to reduce both physical and mental fatigue. The objective is to conserve functional energy so the evening is not marked by such severe exhaustion that family shared time is less compromised.

b. *Establish a Gradual Wind-Down Program and Regular Bedtime*
Patients should relax and do quiet activities for an hour before bedtime. If they do not fall asleep in forty-five minutes, they should get up for awhile.

c. *Keep Their Bedroom as a "Worry Free Zone"*
Encourage patients to leave their worries outside the bedroom and consider their bedroom as their sanctuary away from everyday stresses.

d. *Establish a Sleep Environment That Is Conducive to Sleep*
Patients' sleeping environment should be dark and quiet and they should consider eye-shades and/or earplugs if necessary. Encourage them not to read, watch television or eat in bed.

e. *Keep Their Body Warm*
Patients should be encouraged to take a hot bath or shower before bed and wear a sweat suit and socks in bed if they are cold. They can warm their bed with a hot water bottle or a couple of two-liter pop bottles filled with hot water [Appendix 12].

f. *Support Their Body*
The patients' mattress and pillow should be supportive but not too hard. A contoured pillow for the head and neck, a pillow between the legs and under the top arm help keep the spine in proper alignment and alleviate pain. Tempur-Pedic® mattresses, contoured cervical and lumbar pillows are made from a unique material that was developed for the NASA space program to provide ultimate pressure relief. These products

adapt to and support the body and are approved by Health Canada as Class I medical devices for arthritis, muscular pain, back pain, rheumatism, etc.

g. *Consider Sleep Medication*
Some patients may require sleep medication.

4. *Balanced Diet*
Patients should be encouraged to

a. *Eat at Regular Times*
b. *Eat a Balanced, Nutritious Diet*
Patients who are tired and in chronic pain may require higher nutrient intake to encourage the healing process. Pain reduction and energy enhancement may be achieved in selected patients with a nutritional program of lowered carbohydrates, adequate monounsaturated lipids, and adequate protein in every meal. Patients with hypoglycemia may benefit from food low on the glycemic index. Patients should avoid food to which they are sensitive or aggravates pain.
c. *Drink Enough Water to Keep the Body Well-Hydrated*
d. *Other Nutritional Considerations*

- *Multi-enzyme tablets:* Patients who test low for digestive enzymes may benefit from taking a replacement regimen. A common example is lactose intolerance treated with lactase tablets or enzyme treated milk products.
- *Nutritional supplements* are discussed under "G. Supplements and Herbs." It should be noted that these remedies are seldom documented to be of therapeutic benefit for people with FMS.

5. *Appropriate Body Movement and Fitness*

a. *Patients should be taught good body mechanic habits for lifting, sitting, standing, etc. [Appendix 14].*
b. *Patients should be encouraged to stay as active in their daily activities as they can, within their limits, to maintain strength.*
c. *Patients should avoid heavy work until they have been prepared for it by systematic physical conditioning.*
d. *Patients should be encouraged to adopt and maintain an appropriate exercise program [Appendix 16].*

D. Self-Powered FMS Exercise Programs

Exercise is the most commonly prescribed non-pharmaceutical treatment for FMS and warrants special attention. A systematic review (47) of 1,808 abstracts of multi-disciplinary programs found seven relevant studies that met inclusion criteria for methodology, of which four were for FMS (48-51) and two of those included exercise (48,51). The effectiveness of these studies, as determined by the reviews, was generally disappointing and failed to provide a clear direction for treatment. There is no reliable evidence to explain why exercise should reduce FMS pain (52). Jones et al. (53) reviewed the results of 26 studies on exercise intervention programs involving over 1,200 FMS patients. Some studies indicated improvement but the outcomes were also generally disappointing and did not provide a uniform consensus that exercise is beneficial for the FMS patient. The rate of attrition ran as high as 60 percent and 61 percent and some studies did not disclose their attrition rates. These attrition rates and generally disappointing results suggest a number of the programs fell short of meeting the patients' needs.

Jones and Clark (53,54), exercise physiologists who have studied many exercise programs and the pathophysiology of FMS, have developed guidelines for an individualized exercise program that they have found successful for FMS patients. The following is a combination of their guidelines and additional information from the consensus panel:

1. *Goals and Guidelines*
The philosophy of the exercise program is of the utmost importance. The goals and guidelines given at the beginning of the treatment section must be reflected in the exercise program.
2. *Exercise Must Be Specific to the Pathophysiology of FMS*
As much care must be taken in prescribing exercise programs as is in prescribing pharmaceuticals (55). It is essential that the exercises are specific for the physiological pathology of FMS and the exercise intensity is adapted to the patients' individual abilities/limitations.

If ligaments are weakened or over-stretched, they do not provide adequate support for a joint. Whether the joint is hypermobile or restricted, its movement becomes abnormal. Stretching excites the many pain receptors of the ligaments. Pain impulses go to the nerves of regional muscles as well as being transmitted through the spinal column to the brain, causing the muscles to contract. The muscles are anchored to bones by their tendinous origins and insertions and ultimately to the vertebral spine. Contraction of muscles results in restricted joint movement and decreased circulation. Addressing any tight, shortened muscles is an important part of any exercise program as the tighter the muscles are, the lower is their excitability threshold. These muscles are readily activated, even during movements in which they should be silent. According to the Sherrington's law of reciprocal innervation (56), they influence their antagonist in an inhibitory way. Therefore, the muscles that appear "weak" are not weak but are dysfunctional due to muscle contraction and shortening. After the taut muscles are released and stretched, the majority of these muscles have normal strength. The tight muscles play a primary role in pain complaints.

Therefore, a great deal of care must be taken to warm and stretch the tight muscles before trying to strengthen the weakened, inhibited muscles. Muscle tightness develops mainly due to their overuse [overload]. In moderate tightness, the muscle maintains its strength, or the strength is even increased. However a long-lasting tightness results in muscle weakness. Exercise cannot strengthen or heal ligaments and tendons, which are often at the heart of the problem; but will in fact, cause progressive degeneration if their tensile strength is exceeded. Warming muscles and specific stretches will help lengthen taut muscles and reduce stress on the ligaments and joints. *Thus, it is essential to establish a program that avoids worsening the patient's condition and pain (52).*

3. *Initial Patient Evaluation*
A thorough assessment of the patient's history, physical condition, and total illness burden must be made prior to prescribing exercise. *Pain generators and risk factors must be identified.* These include prior injuries, tight shortened muscles, painful myofascial trigger points, lax or injured ligaments and/or tendons, osteoarthritis in weight bearing joints, risk for adverse cardiac events during exercise, balance problems, orthostatic intolerance, problems with eccentric muscle work, and reduced level of fitness. Medication may have a positive or negative effect.

The patient *must* be thoroughly examined for increased muscle tone and concurrent muscle shortening, muscle imbalance, and hypermobile or restricted joints. As many FMS patients also exhibit active or latent MPS trigger points, these should be assessed. Special attention should be given to the connections of the lumbosacral spine where it is joined to the pelvis at the sacroiliac joints as weakened ligaments can allow the sacrum between the iliac bones to become locked in an abnormal position or displaced causing extensive muscle shortening and imbalance. The concept of "myotactic unit" as described in Travell and Simons (57,58), is helpful in organizing muscle examinations.

4. *Optimize Medical Management Prior to Introducing an Exercise Program*
Patients who benefit most from non-fatiguing exercise are those, whose pain and concomitant conditions are under control. Whether or not FMS patients will benefit from exercise depends on many factors such as weakened ligaments or tendons, taut muscles and muscle imbalance, concomitant arthritis or muscle disease, current level of conditioning, appropriateness of exercise, rate of increase of intensity, ratio of eccentric to concentric muscle use, etc. FMS patients who also meet the criteria of myalgic encephalomyelitis/chronic fatigue syndrome have less tolerance for exercise and greater post-exertional malaise and/or fatigue. Ligaments should be strengthened, and taut muscles should be released before the patient does strengthening and endurance exercises. These exercises may not be recommended for some patients.

5. *Principles of a Self-Powered Exercise Program*

The professional must be knowledgeable about the pathophysiology of FMS and utilize the following principles.

a. *Minimize Muscle Microtrauma and Emphasize Low Intensity Exercise*

It is essential that muscles are warmed and stretched out before exercising as exercising chronically taut muscles results in further weakness. The most important factor in keeping the patient active is to use low intensity exercise to avoid microtrauma and overuse of dysfunctional muscles and joints as that will increase the local and generalized pain that often lasts two to five days, and can cause further muscle or ligament damage. Very gradually, over months, increase to a moderate intensity if tolerated. If the exercise produces pain, reduce its intensity. Avoid movements that produce eccentric muscle contractions [the muscle contracts while elongated] such as overhead strength and endurance movements.

b. *Minimize Central Sensitization*

Activities that would be considered trivial to a healthy person can cause pain and injury in FMS patients. Sensory input from overloaded or dysfunctional muscles can activate central sensitization and cause reactive pain, which in turn can lead to patients' avoidance. Help patients find the right level of intensity of exercise to allow them to be active without causing flare-ups.

c. *Maximize Self-Efficacy and Minimize Attrition*

In order for exercises to have the desired effect of having patients maintain function in their daily living activities, patients need to incorporate them into their daily lives. Exercises that cause significant pain and/or worsen the patients' conditions will lead to attrition. Ensure ongoing success by adapting exercises to patients' abilities/limitations. It is essential that patients have a sense of autonomy.

6. *Write an Individualized Exercise Program in Conjunction with the Patient*

FMS patients are not a homogeneous group. A "one size fits all" exercise program does not work. *An individualized exercise program must be tailored to the specific patient.*

It is important to allow patients to express their expectations and concerns so that the exercise program is adapted to accommodate their circumstances and needs. Always begin the program at the patient's base level of conditioning and take into account that FMS patients experience more post-exertional pain and amplification of sensory processing (59,60). It is helpful to have patients keep a checklist of exercises and daily activities that they can do without exacerbating pain. Have patients take their temperature before and after exercise. If temperature drops after exercising, they have done too much. *Patients should be encouraged to "listen to their body" and stop before they are in pain.* The program should include the following components:

a. *Warm-Up and Warm-Down Periods*

These periods are important to prevent muscle injury and pain. Patients should be encouraged to have a hot bath or shower, or use hot packs before stretching because the warmer their muscles, the easier and less painful they are to stretch.

b. *Stretching*

Stretching is essential. When performed properly, stretching can loosen up tight, shortened muscles and relieve pain in the tightened muscle bands. Breathing techniques while stretching are most important. Patients should breathe in and then *as* they breathe *out*, they should stretch to the point of resistance and hold the stretch for a few seconds. Holding the stretch will "allow the Golgi tendon apparatus to signal the muscle fibers to relax" (54). Patients should begin by holding a stretch at the point of resistance and then *very gently and gradually* increase the stretch range by increasing the number of breathing and stretching cycles *within their limits*. Patients must avoid stretching muscles to the point of pain as that will cause additional fibers to contract.

c. *Strength Training*

Tight muscles must be warmed and stretched prior to any strengthening exercise. Exercises and stretches must be specific to each patient and each muscle group or the patient's condition and pain may worsen. Strengthening muscles and stabilizing joints enables the patient to do daily activities and improve her/his health. The focus is on muscle toning and functional strength and should include exercises to improve the strength of the upper and lower body, abdominal and paraspinal areas. Exercises should accommodate for the delay in the muscles returning to a resting state following a muscle contraction in FMS patients (61). For example, when doing a bicep curl, the patient begins by sitting on a chair with arms resting on the lap, moving the fist up to the shoulder [4 counts], returning the arms down to beginning position [2 counts] and relaxing [4-8 counts]. Sit-ups are not recommended as they may result in contracture of the hip flexors [rectus femoris and iliopsoas], rather than the abdominal muscles. Remind the patient to keep movements on a parallel plane and minimize eccentric movements that can cause microtrauma and pain, such as overhead strength and endurance movements.

d. *Endurance Conditioning*

These exercises should be non-impact loading. Have patients find activities that they find enjoyable, such as walking at a comfortable pace or gentle acquacise in a heated pool. For those patients who are limited in their ability to walk, exercise can be done while sitting on a chair.

e. *Balance*

Alterations in sensory and motor functions can affect balance. Light intensity exercise can improve balance. [See appendix 14 for how to establish center of balance.]

f. *Pacing*

Jones and Clark have found that the best results are obtained by pacing in the fol-

lowing manner, which can be used as a guideline:

- *Stretching* can be done a number of times a day.
- *Strength training:* A warm-up and warm-down period and stretching must be done before any strengthening exercise, e.g., day 1–upper body, day 2–no strength training, day 3–lower body, day 4–no strength training, and then repeat cycle.
- *Endurance:* Start with 3 minutes and gradually increase as tolerated. Some patients may find it better to gradually work up to two or three short walks than one long one.
- *Strengthening and endurance exercises do not need to be done at the same time or in the same day.*

It is most important that patients have a sense of control over the pacing of their exercise program. The *intensity* and *duration* of the exercises should be adapted to the patients' abilities. If an exercise causes pain, reduce the intensity before reducing the frequency. Encourage patients to decrease the time and intensity on bad days but not to overdo it on good days. Patients should end their exercise sessions feeling they could do a little more (53,54). *Self-powered success leads to continued commitment and success!*

See Appendix 16 for examples of stretches and exercises appropriate for FMS patients.

E. Pharmacological Treatments

NOTE: This is NOT a systematic review of available pharmacological treatments. The following is an overview of some of the medications, which members of the panel have found helpful for some patients in their clinical practice.

[This is NOT an endorsement for any commercial product.]

Therapeutic Principles

1. Keep the therapeutic regimen as simple, effective, and inexpensive as possible.

2. Many patients with FMS are unusually sensitive to medication given in the usual doses.

Always start at a lower dose than recommended, and gradually build up to ensure tolerance. Add or subtract remedies one at a time, and give remedies enough time to show their effects beyond non-specific "placebo" effects [approximately 3 months]. Keep testing medications by withdrawing them to see if they are still necessary, and using N = 1 trials if indicated. [See Appendix 11.] Caution is advised regarding the addictive potential of benzodiazepines and narcotic analgesics.

3. The plethora of these remedies shows that none are universally effective.

Many remedies help a few patients to varying degrees, but none help all of them. Trial and error and lack of side effects can determine the effectiveness of a remedy for an individual patient.

4. Level of Evidence [LE] Categories

   I. Large double blind randomized, control trials [RCTs], or meta-analyses of smaller RCTs, clinically relevant outcomes

   II. Small RCTs, non-blinded RCTs, RCTs using valid surrogate markers

   III. Non-randomized controlled studies, observational [cohort] studies, case-control studies, or cross-sectional studies

   IV. Opinion of expert committees or respected authorities

   V. Expert opinion

   VI. Unsupported clinical opinion

   VII. Shown to be no better than placebo

Where possible, the level of evidence is indicated. There have been few blind-controlled studies on pharmaceuticals for FMS. Therefore, many of the recommendations and therapies have not been subjected to strict clinical trials or may not have been scientifically duplicated/confirmed. However, they are mentioned because there is some evidence and scientific basis for their inclusion. The recommendations of experts in the field with clinical experience justifies their inclusion and are still worth pursuing as their value may be confirmed in the future. The clinician should be most influenced to try medications for the treatment of FMS symptoms if the medication is supported by "levels of evidence" [LE] I to III.

Pharmaceuticals

The primary source of information of the tables concerning more common and important side effects is the clinical experience of the expert panel members. This has been supplemented by information from the *Compendium of Pharmaceuticals and Specialties*, 36 edition 2001, Canadian Pharmacist's Association (*www. intilihealth.com*) for new drugs; and *Herbs: Everyday Reference for Health Professionals*, editor in chief, Frank Chandler, 200, Canadian Pharmacist Association and Canadian Medical Association; and individual references as sited.

The panel ranked the following pharmaceuticals in logical order, taking into account the number of members of the panel favoring the pharmaceutical and its variance. Different patients are helped by different pharmaceuticals. Clinical judgment is advised.

1. *Pain*

Pharmaceuticals for Pain	
NOTE: "LE" and Roman numeral at the end of comments, stands for "level of evidence," "+" indicates positive effects, and "±" indicates mixed effects.	
Pharmaceutical	Dose/Effects/Comments
a. *Non-Narcotic Analgesics*	
Acetaminophen	325 mg tablets 1-2 PO q4h prn. Use as baseline analgesic therapy. Weak effect, but low incidence of side effects. LE I: ± results. Synergistic with tramadol, cariprodol (62,63).

b. *NSAID [Nonsteroidal Anti-Inflammatories]*	
Watch for GI side-effects, especially GI bleeding, as well as hepatic dysfunction, renal dysfunction, peripheral edema, CNS side effects such as headache, dizziness, drowsiness and evidence of hypersensitivity. Use NSAID precautions to prevent GI side effects.	
Ibuprofen	200 mg qid prn LE II, VI, VII: ± results. The results are inadequately beneficial as a monotherapy, but it works synergistically with alprazolam (64,65).
Naproxen	250 mg tid prn. Longer acting than ibuprofen. LE II, VI, VII: ± results. The results are inadequately beneficial as a monotherapy, but it works synergistic with amitriptyline (66,67).
c. *COX-2 Inhibitors: [Cyclooxygenase-2]*	
Side effects commonly come from the GI tract and CNS and include dyspepsia, abdominal pain, nausea, constipation, diarrhea, flatulence, peptic ulcers, gastrointestinal bleeding, headache, dizziness, and somnolence. Watch for hypersensitivity reactions. Use NSAID precautions. Not recommended for long-term use.	
Celecoxib	100 mg bid LE V: ± results. May be safer than NSAIDs. No studies for FMS (68).
Rofecoxib	12.5-25 mg daily LE V: ± results. May be safer than NSAIDs. No studies for FMS (68).
d. *TCA: [Tricyclic Antidepressants]*	
"Start low, go slow." Low dose tricyclic antidepressants may be effective for some patients in the *short-term. Patients should be warned of typical weight gain.* Dry mouth, and morning grogginess are common at onset. Watch for daytime sedation, difficulty concentrating, cognitive dysfunction, nausea, sleep disturbance, dizziness, headache, and weakness. Benefits are usually seen within *2 to 4 weeks.* Reassess frequently for effect/side-effect balance.	
Amitriptyline	5-100 mg. Start with lowest dose qhs and gradually increase to effective dose schedule, splitting the dose (69). LE I: ± results. Most studied drug in FMS (67,70-81).
Doxepin	5-100 mg qhs as tolerated LE V: ± results. Used in FMS but inadequately studied (76).
Cyclobenzaprine	Up to 10 mg tid as tolerated. Tricyclic skeletal muscle relaxant. LE I: + results. Comparable to amitriptyline (70,82-86).
e. *SSRIs: [Selective Serotonin Reuptake Inhibitors]*	
Always start with lowest dose and gradually increase as tolerated. Common side effects include faintness, palpitations, increased sweating, nausea, trembling, headaches, dry mouth, diarrhea, constipation, drowsiness, difficulty sleeping, paresthesia, anorexia, and male sexual dysfunction. They have a lower frequency of anticholinergic, sedating and cardiovascular side effects than TCAs but may cause more gastrointestinal complaints, sleep impairment, and sexual dysfunction.	
Fluoxetine	5-20 mg qod as tolerated LE II: ± results. Effective alone for depression in normal dosage, effective for pain only in high dose [40-60 mg/d], synergistic in low dose with amitriptyline (77,87,88).
f. *Anti-Convulsants/GABA Receptor Agonist*	
For pain with neuropathic features. Watch for initial side effects of sedation.	

Gabapentin	Build up to 100 mg bid-900 mg tid. Sometimes helpful for severe pain in high doses [3,600 mg/d in divided doses]. Structurally related to the neurotransmitter GABA, but of uncertain mode of action. Described as an anti-epileptic and approved for refractory partial seizures. Effects may also include improved sleep, increased energy, reduced anxiety, and depression (89, p. 144). More common side effects include fatigue, somnolence, dizziness, ataxia, nystagmus, tremor, rhinitis, and peripheral edema. LE V: + results. Used with benefit in high dosage but inadequately studied (90-92).
g. *Local Anesthetics*	
Lidocaine	IV 5 mg/kg over 30 min. Beneficial effect may last several days. LE II, III: ± results. Effective for some FMS patients when given IM or by vein, not when given in skin or sphenopalatine ganglion (93-97).
h. *Needling and Injections Therapies:* See Alternative/Complementary Approaches in following section.	
i. *Neurotransmitter Precursors*	
5-Hydroxy tryptophan [5-HTP]	Being with 100 mg daily. Increase dose during day to achieve pain control and dose at qhs for sleep. The daily dose varies considerably, but upper limit [not defined] is probably 500-600 mg. Side effects include nausea, headaches, and agitation. LE II: + results. Low level in the brain of FMS patients, effective Rx (98,99).
j. *Narcotics*	
Patients with severe pain may need narcotics. The use of narcotics requires a clear rationale with documentation which is difficult when no clinical studies support their use for FMS. They are only to be used if other treatments fail. Use with caution based on risk versus benefit. Use standard dosage and increase in dosage or potency for adequate pain control. *Abuse potential: alert patient to habituating nature of these drugs.*	
Codeine	15-60 mg. Major hazards associated with codeine are respiratory and CNS depression. More common side effects include sedation, nausea and vomiting, constipation, light-headedness, dizziness, and sweating. LE V: + results. No studies, dependency risk.
Vicodin, Fentanyl patch, Long acting MS, methadone	There are no placebo-controlled clinical studies to support the use of these drugs for the treatment of pain in people with FMS. [MS = morphine sulfate] LE V, VI: ± results, physical dependency expected.
k. *Others*	
Tramadol	5-10 mg. Available by special release. LE I: + results. Effective, mild μ-opioid agonist but not principally a narcotic because the main effects are believed to come from concomitant biogenic amine uptake inhibition (63,100-102).
Baclofen	5-20 mg tid as tolerated. Mode of action is uncertain but probably acts as a GABA-B agonist. Listed as a muscle relaxant and antispastic. It also has an effect on central pain, is an anxiolytic, and may cause increased alertness (89). Side effects include drowsiness, fatigue, dizziness, weakness, headache, insomnia, hypertension, nausea, constipation, urinary frequency, and muscular myotonia. LE V: No studies involving FMS.

Ketamine	At least two groups of investigators (103-107) have tested ketamine in FMS. It antagonizes the effects of the excitatory amino acids at the NMDA receptor. It seems to be effective in reducing the severity of the pain in a subgroup [50 percent] of FMS patients but not in all (103,104). A problem with this agent is that the drug often induces adverse effects before it reaches a therapeutic concentration and when the agent administration is discontinued, the therapeutic effect is lost before the adverse effects fully resolve. LE 1: Small controlled studies.

2. Fatigue

Pharmaceuticals for Fatigue	
NOTE: "LE" and Roman numeral at the end of comments, stands for "level of evidence," "+" indicates positive effects, and "±" indicates mixed effects.	
Drug	*Dose/Effects/Comments*
a. *Antiepileptic*	
See discussion under pain for further side effects.	
Gabapentin	100 mg bid-300 mg tid. Start with low dose, and increase gradually as tolerated. Pain control benefit may require 3,600mg/day. Note: with lessening of fatigue, there is a tendency to push beyond activity boundaries, with resultant exacerbation of symptoms. LE V: + results. Used with benefit in high dosage but inadequately studied (90-92)
b. *Others*	
Cyanocobalamin	Draw baseline serum B12 and red cell folate [best taken in AM]. If B12 is low, start with B12 at 1000 mcg once per week parenterally. In two weeks increase dose to 1000 mcg twice weekly. Increase dose by 1000 mcg every two weeks until the maximum dose of 2000 to 3000 mcg every 2-3 days is achieved. It is recommended that those who do not respond well take 1 mg of folic acid daily in tablet form. To prevent deficiencies of other B complex vitamins, it is recommended that patients supplement their daily diet with multi-vitamins containing B-complex and folic acid. Note: oral and sublingual B12 are usually ineffective. Discontinue if no improvement is seen within 3 months. LE V: No studies in FMS.
Venlafaxine	18.75 mg qAM, then increase to 37.5 mg bid. Maximum daily dose should not exceed 150 mg. LE III: ± results. Uncertain benefit in some (101,108,109).
DHEA	Use only for a confirmed DHEA sulfate deficiency. [Presently one needs to apply for special authorization from Health Canada on an individual patient basis for the use of DHEA. The product used in this program is pure.] In the USA, it is recommended that DHEA be obtained from a compounding pharmacy because over-the counter preparations vary widely in purity and amount of actual DHEA present in the product. LE V: No studies in FMS.

Pyridostigmine	60 mg twice daily, and increase cautiously, as tolerated. Do not crush tablet. It is a cholinergic agent to enhance the transmission of impulses across neuromuscular junctions. May counteract somatostatin inhibition of growth hormone release during aerobic exercise. Side effects include salivation, muscular fasciculation, abdominal cramps, and diarrhea. LE II: + results. Facilitated exercise-induced growth hormone production in FMS (110,111).

3. *Sleep Disturbance*

The exact cause of the sleep disturbance should be determined. Consider both the sleep quantity and its quality of being restorative or not. Early insomnia may be simply due to restlessness and may respond to mild sedatives. Adequate pain control medication and often muscle relaxants best manage interruption of sleep by pain. Terminal insomnia is usually due to intrinsic anxiety or depression and is best treated by anti-depressants. Restless legs syndrome may respond to anticonvulsants, clonazepam, or carbidopa/levodopa. Awakening due to paresthesia should be managed by attention to neck support during sleep. Patients on long-term therapy should be assessed periodically.

It has been reported (112) that as many as 40 percent of male FMS patients have sleep apnea, which should be investigated. Surgery or an intermittent positive pressure-breathing device can be helpful for many people with the obstructive form (113-115), while pacing the diaphragm can be helpful in the idiopathic central form (116).

Pharmaceuticals for Sleep Disturbance	
NOTE: "LE" and Roman numeral at the end of comments, stands for "level of evidence," "+" indicates positive effects, and "±" indicates mixed effects.	
Drug	*Dose/Effects/Comments*
a. *Hypnotics*	
Zopiclone	3.75-7.5 mg qhs. It may increase amount of stage III and IV sleep. Effect lasts up to 7 hours. Side effects to watch for include excessive drowsiness, incoordination, and early morning bitter taste in mouth. LE II: + results. Effective but rebound is a problem (117-119).
b. *Tricyclic Antidepressants*	
"Start low, go slow." Often effective for sleep in the *short term. Warn about possible weight gain. Side effects can be significant even at low dose*–especially early morning grogginess and confusion, dry mouth, increased appetite, constipation, urinary retention, blurred vision, palpitations, hypotension. Reassess patient periodically. Side effects are often dose related and if tolerated, tend to decrease with time. Benefits are usually seen 2-4 weeks after initiation. *Do not use in the presence of monoamine oxidase [MAO] inhibitors. Tricyclics may enhance the effects of alcohol and other CNS depressants.*	
Amitriptyline	5-10 mg qhs to start; gradually increase by 10 mg qhs until optimal effect [20–50 mg] if tolerated. Tachyphylaxis responds to a month-long drug holiday every three to four months. LE I: + results. Most studied drug in FMS (67,70-81).
Doxepin	10-75 mg qhs LE V: ± results. Used in FMS but inadequate study (120).
Cyclobenzaprine	Up to 10 mg tid as tolerated. 10 mg qhs. For short-term use, reassess periodically. LE I: + results. Comparable to amitriptyline (67,70,82-85).

c. *Benzodiazepines*	
The common side effects are related to CNS depression; especially drowsiness, inco-ordination and ataxia. *Patients must be cautioned that benzodiazepines can be highly addictive.*	
Clonazepam	0.5-2 mg qhs. It is an intermediate onset of action [1-3 hours] for sleep induction, and is often used in combination with Doxepin to obtain both rapid and prolonged effects on sleep. It may be helpful for *nocturnal myoclonus.* LE III: + results. Beneficial in nocturnal myoclonus (121-123).
Oxazepam	15-30 mg qhs. LE V: no studies involving FMS.
d. *Polycyclics*	
Common side effects include excessive drowsiness, nausea, headache, and dry mouth. Also watch for less common manifestations of CNS depression, cardiac arrhythmias and postural hypotension, constipation, urinary retention, priapism, and allergic manifestations. Precautions are similar to those for tricyclics.	
Trazodone	25-100 mg qhs. It is a tetracyclic sedative and antidepressant. It increases the depth and quality of sleep. Substitute for amitriptyline when side effects are too limiting. LE III: + results. Uncontrolled observation only (124,125).
e. *Muscle Relaxants*	
Cyclobenzaprine	10 mg qhs. Tricyclic skeletal muscle relaxant. LE I: + results. See tricyclic antidepressants above.
Tizanidine	4 mg q 6-8 h as tolerated. Increase dose as tolerated. Total maximum daily dose is not to exceed 36 mg. For cramps, pain, and sleep. Common side effects include dry mouth, sleepiness, tiredness, weakness, and dizziness. LE III: + results. Clinically effective and decreased spinal fluid substance P (126,127).
Baclofen	5-20 mg tid as tolerated. See Baclofen under Pain. LE V: No studies for FMS.
Carisoprodol	350 mg qhs-tid Concern about dependency. Side effects from the CNS include drowsiness, dizziness, tremor, headache, depression, and insomnia. A variety of allergic or idiosyncratic reactions may be seen. Cardiovascular side effects include tachycardia, hypotension, and facial flushing. GI side effects include nausea, vomiting, hiccup, and indigestion. LE II: + results. Effective in combinations (62,128).
f. *Nocturnal Myoclonus [Periodic Leg Movement Syndrome]*	
Clonazepam	0.5-2 mg qhs A benzodiazepine. See effects/side effects under sleep. LE III: + results. Beneficial in nocturnal myoclonus but no studies in FMS (121-123).

Pergolide	0.05 mg once daily for 2 days, then increase by 0.1 mg as tolerated. Maintenance dose administration is 3 times daily, maximum dose is 5 mg daily. A dopamine agonist. Side effects include dyskinesia, dizziness, hallucinations, somnolence, and insomnia. There may also be nausea, constipation, diarrhea, postural hypertension, and respiratory problems including rhinitis. LE II: + results. Beneficial for nocturnal myoclonus (129).
Carbidopa/ levodopa	Start with 100/10 mg tid-qid. Side effects include involuntary movements, nausea, cardiac irregularities, orthostatic hypotension, hallucinations, confusion, dizziness, headache, depression, somnolence, and asthenia. Rarely gastrointestinal bleeding, anemia, thrombocytopenia, leukopenia sand agranulocytosis may occur. *Some patients are very sensitive to it so doses must be tailored.* LE II, V: ± results. No studies (129).
g. *Others*	
5-hydroxy- tryptophan [5-HTP]	Start 10 mg tid-20 mg qhs. Upper limit ~500 mg per day [not defined]. Increase doses during the day to achieve pain control and dose at hs to achieve improved sleep. It is usually used in conjunction with L-dopa ± carbidopa. Carbidopa blocks the enzyme that converts 5-HTP to serotonin, so carbidopa inhibits the serotonergic effects of 5-HTP. *Some patients are exquisitely sensitive to this agent. Doses must be much smaller for these patients.* Antispastic agent, alpha adrenergic agonist. Side effects include dry mouth, somnolence, asthenia, dizziness, urinary tract infection, constipation, hypotension, and bradycardia. LE II: + results. Low level in the brain of FMS patients, effective RX (98,99). Studied effective dosage was 100 mg TID.

4. *Other Comorbid Symptoms*

Dizziness: Simple instructions to avoid neck extension or quick rotation may be sufficient if dizziness is caused by proprioceptive disturbances in the neck.

Pharmaceuticals for Other Comorbid Symptoms	
NOTE: "LE" and Roman numeral at the end of comments, stands for "level of evidence," "+" indicates positive effects, and "±" indicates mixed effects.	
Neurally Mediated Hypotension [NMH]	
NMH, a positional paradoxical hypotensive response, should be confirmed with a tilt-table test before beginning trials of therapy. Always begin with non-medical interventions. [See appendix 13.] Start by increasing salt intake with adequate water intake. Consider fludrocortisone [for blood volume expansion] if the salt seems to help for a while but then loses its effectiveness. One may also add an alpha 1 agonist [vasoconstrictor agent], such as midodrine.	
Drug	*Dose/Effects/Comments*
Fludrocortisone	0.05-0.2 mg daily. Increases sodium and water retention and may inhibit vasodilation. As it is a mineralocorticosteroid, be careful to monitor serum potassium levels and use the minimal effective dose. Side effects are extension of its effects–excessive fluid retention, potassium loss, and hypertension. LE II: ± results. Used in ME/CFS, no studies in FMS (130-133).

Midodrine	Start at 2.5 mg tid, increasing to 5 mg tid if tolerated. It is an alpha-adrenergic agonist. Side effects include supine hypertension, palpitations, headache, bradycardia, pruritus, and urinary retention. It can be used in conjunction with fludrocortisone since the mechanism of action is different. LE II: + results. No studies in FMS (134).

Vertigo

Vertigo accompanied by nystagmus, nausea, and/or vomiting is often associated with tinnitus, and/or impaired hearing acuity. An anti-nauseant may give partial relief.

Meclozine	25 mg daily, increasing to 25 mg tid. An antiemetic with antihistaminic and anticholinergic properties. Side effects include drowsiness, fatigue and dry mouth. LE II: + results. Equal to scopolamine patch for vertigo, no experience with FMS (135).

Nocturnal Myoclonus [Restless Legs Syndrome] Above Under Sleep Disturbance

Irritable Bowel Syndrome

Watch for food intolerance and conduct food elimination trials.

Pinaverium	50 mg tid prn. Efficacy uncertain. Gastrointestinal calcium antagonist. Side effects include mild gastrointestinal disturbances, headaches, dry mouth, drowsiness, and vertigo. LE I: + results. Beneficial in IBS. No studies in FMS (136-145).
Hyoscine	10 mg tid prn. An anticholinergic antispasmodic. Side effects are extensions of its effects including dry mouth, dyshidrosis, visual accommodation disturbances, tachycardia, dyspnea, urinary retention, dizziness, hypotension, and hypersensitivity reactions. LE I: + results. Beneficial in IBS. No studies in FMS (141-148).
Mebervine	One sachet [135 mg] bid to tid. Side effects are depression, headaches, dizziness, diarrhea, and constipation. LE I: + results. Beneficial in IBS. No studies in FMS (137,141).

Bladder Dysfunction: Interstitial Cystitis Syndrome [ICS]

Oxybutynin	5 mg tid prn. A tertiary amine anticholinergic antispasmotic. Side effects are similar to those of hyoscine and also include syncope, weakness, headaches, nausea, vomiting, constipation, and hypersensitivity reactions. LE II: + results. Instilled directly into the bladder. Beneficial in ICS (149).
Flavoxate	200 mg tid prn. Papaverine-like smooth muscle relaxant. Side effects include nausea, vomiting, dry mouth, increased ocular tension [use with caution in patients with glaucoma], blurred vision, skin rashes, jaundice, mental confusion, palpitations, and tachycardia. Rare cases of sudden death in older patients. LE II: + results. Not studied in FMS or ICS (150-156).

Anxiety	
a. Benzodiazepines	
Common side effects are the result of CNS depression including drowsiness, over-sedation, impairment of cognition and psychomotor performance, ataxia, and behavioral disturbances. Also watch for nausea, constipation, diarrhea and rashes. *Cautions for all benzodiazepines: potential for tolerance, dependence and abuse. Regularly reassess need. Always reduce medication very gradually to minimize withdrawal reactions.*	
Alprazolam	0.125 mg bid to max. of 2 mg in divided doses. LE I, II: + results. Anxiolytic. In FMS it is beneficial in synergy with ibuprofen (121,157).
Clonazepam	0.5 mg daily to 0.5 mg tid. LE I, II: + results. Anxiolytic. Beneficial in nocturnal myoclonus. No studies in FMS (121-123).
Diazepam	2-5 mg 3-4 times daily. LE I, II: + results. Anxiolytic. Possibly beneficial in IC with FMS (158).
Lorazepam	0.5 mg daily to 1.0 mg bid. LE I, II: + results. Anxiolytic. One reference to FMS (100).
Oxazepam	10 mg daily to 10-15 mg tid. LE I, II: + results. Anxiolytic. No reference to FMS.
b. Others	
Buspirone	5 mg 2-3 times daily to max. of 20 mg daily in divided doses. It is an azaspirone with clinical similarity to benzodiazepines. This should not be used with MAO inhibitors. It is non-sedating and does not lead to tolerance or dependence. Side effects include dizziness, headaches, nervousness, light-headedness, nausea, anorexia, and sweating. LE I, II: + results. No reference to FMS.
Depression	
a. SSRIs	
First line choice for treatment of depression. Note: they are not usually effective in treating fatigue and may interfere with sleep. They have a lower frequency of anticholinergic, sedating, and cardiovascular side effects than the TCAs but possibly cause more gastrointestinal complaints, sleep impairment, and sexual dysfunction. Side effects include headache, nervousness, insomnia, somnolence, anxiety, fatigue, tremor, dizziness, nausea, diarrhea, anorexia, dry mouth, excessive sweating, and allergic reactions. Do not use in close temporal proximity to MAO inhibitors.	
Fluoxetine	5-20 mg daily max. 40 mg daily. LE II: + results. Effective alone for depression. Reduces pain only in high dose, synergistic in low dose with amitriptyline (77,87,88,159).
Sertraline	25-100 mg with evening meal. There is perhaps a lower risk of drug interactions than with the other SSRIs. LE II: ? results. No traditional efficacy studies in FMS (81,160,161).
Citalopram	5-40 mg daily qAM or pm, max. 40 mg daily. LE II: + results. Persistent benefit on depression, transient benefit on pain and well-being (162).
Paroxetine	5-10 mg daily qAM, going to 20 mg daily, max. 40 mg daily. More anticholinergic side effects than fluoxetine or sertraline. LE I: + results. Effective in depression. No studies in FMS (163).

Fluvoxamine	5-40 mg LE I: + results. Effective in depression. No studies in FMS (164,165).
b. *TCA*	
They are not first line choices for *antidepressant effects* because many side effects occur at the dose required. *Note: Most FMS patients cannot tolerate a dose high enough to get the antidepressant effect. Advise patients of possible weight gain.* Watch for antihistaminic side effects [sedation] and anticholinergic side effects [constipation, dry mouth, urinary hesitancy, and blurred vision]. Watch for cardiovascular side effects of orthostatic hypotension, tachycardia, arrhythmias; confusional states, agitation, insomnia, ataxia, nausea, allergic manifestations. *Watch for drug interaction and do not use in close temporal proximity to MAO inhibitors.*	
Amitriptyline	5 mg hs Gradually increase to 100 mg daily as tolerated. Keep dose on low side. LE I: + results. Antidepressant in higher dosage than used for FMS management.
Nortriptyline	Start at 10 mg. Gradually increase to 50-100 mg daily as tolerated. Side effects are similar to but usually fewer and less severe than with amitriptyline. LE I: + results. Antidepressant. No studies in FMS.
Imipramine	Start at 10 mg hs. Gradually increase to 100 mg daily as tolerated. Side effects include dry mouth and early morning sedation. LE I: + results. Antidepressant. No studies in FMS.
Doxepin	Start at 5-10 mg hs. Gradually increase to 75-100 mg daily in divided doses as tolerated. LE I: + results. Antidepressant. No studies in FMS.
c. *Other*	
Bupropion	Start at 100 mg sustained release once daily, going to 150 mg daily as tolerated. An aminoketone with noradrenergic function. It has no anticholinergic sedating or orthostatic side effects, but may have aversive stimulant-like side effects. Other side effects include headache, agitation, anxiety, insomnia, rashes, dry mouth, nausea, and rhinitis. A rare serum sickness-like reaction has been reported. *Do not use in close temporal proximity to MAO inhibitors.* LE I, II: + results. No reference to FMS.

Target Therapy of FMS. It is anticipated that the optimal therapy for FMS in the near future will be established using a limited cocktail of low-dose medications, which each target a specific receptor known to be involved in the pathogenesis of FMS. By keeping the dosages below the usual toxicity level for each and choosing agents with different kinds of toxicity, it may be possible to achieve clinical benefit while avoiding toxicity.

E. Alternative/Complementary Approaches

Traditional and non-traditional, non-pharmacological treatments are commonly used for FMS. In many cases their effectiveness is based on anecdotal reports. It should be emphasized that the majority of non-traditional non-prescription treatments do not have evidence-based data to confirm their effectiveness. Physicians are aware that many of their FMS patients seek out non-traditional, non-prescription treatments because the standard treatments have not provided significant benefits for symptoms. Therefore, practicing physicians should be knowledgeable about alternate treatments to promote communication with their patients and integrate other health care providers into the treatment programs.

The following is an overview of various non-traditional and/or non-pharmaceutical therapeutic practices. These treatments require specialized training. Their effectiveness is mainly anecdotal and highly variable. No known therapy helps all patients but some are helpful for some patients. [This is not an endorsement for any commercial product or intervention concept.]

1. *Needling and Injection Therapies*
   Good results of needling and injection therapies require a correct diagnosis, excellent knowledge of muscle and functional anatomy, extensive training in the form of workshops and apprenticeships, and practice.

   a. *Prolotherapy*
   If there is benign laxity in ligamentous tissue or it is forcibly stretched by trauma, the ligament is unable to return to its normal length. Thus, it becomes lax and allows the joint to move beyond its normal range of motion. Sensory nerves become irritated and will produce local and referred chronic pain, numbness and/or tingling. Muscles will contract in an attempt to stabilize the joint and protect it from further damage. There is a tendency to treat the muscle spasms and pain rather than the ligament strain or tear, which may be the primary cause. Contracted muscles usually release when the ligaments are strengthened in such cases.
   Prolotherapy (166) [Proliferative, Reconstructive Therapy or previously known as Sclerotherapy] is claimed to be effective for the repair of loose or torn ligaments. A proliferative agent, of which there are over 250 [the simplest being hyperosmotic Dextrose 15-17 percent], is mixed with a local anesthetic such as lidocaine or procaine [or without] and using an appropriate needle and syringe, it is then injected into the fibro-osseous junction of the damaged ligament. This results in a locally directed inflammatory response and the subsequent stimulation of the fibroblast to make new collagen, which provides thickening and strengthening of ligaments. The new fibrous or

ligamentous tissue is said to result in "repair" of this area. As this is a local, controlled reaction, it may be repeated as often as necessary [usually 1-4 times] and to all areas which require this therapy.
   While prolotherapy is still considered an experimental treatment due to insufficient controlled studies, it has been used successfully for pain relief from ligament laxity for approximately sixty years and has demonstrated long-lasting results. In a study by Reeves (167), prolotherapy reduced the pain levels and increased functional abilities in more than 75 percent of severe FMS patients.

Prolotherapy does remarkably well at eliminating the pain caused by ligament relaxation or weakness.

> *. . . C. Everett Koop, M.D.*
> *former US Surgeon General (21)*

   b. *Intramuscular Stimulation or "Dry Needling" of MPS Trigger Points [TrPs]*
   When muscles with MPS are found in FMS patients this method may help. Dry Needling is more correctly referred to as "Intramuscular Stimulation" (168). This technique utilizes an acupuncture needle of varying diameter and length, within a manual Japanese needle plunger, allowing the needle to be inserted any number of times into TrPs or taut fibrotic bands, to allow the muscle to relax and lengthen. This thin needle also allows sensitive feedback concerning the consistencies of the tissues penetrated.

   c. *Myofascial Trigger Point Injection*
   Another technique used to relax and lengthen taut fibrotic bands is TrP injection. This technique is explained and delineated by Travell and Simons (57). Their textbooks are suggested reading for anyone who may be interested in exploring this form of therapy. In its simplest form, TrP Injection consists of localizing the tight taut band and the trigger point in the muscle in question. Pressure over the TrP should reproduce the patient's pain and referral pattern as outlined in their text. The spot of most

tenderness and referral is then injected percutaneously with dilute [0.5 percent] Xylocaine or Procaine [without] using an appropriate needle usually 25 gauge to 30 gauge in 1/2 to 2 inch lengths and syringes. The amount injected depends on the size of the muscle and its TrP as well as the practitioner's proficiency–usually 0.1 ml to 3 ml. Concurrent with the injection, the muscle will usually contract then release and lengthen [which may be visible], then reproduce the patient's pain and referral pattern. This may provide temporary relief. It should be noted that TrP injection therapy is less successful for MPS when it occurs in the setting of FMS than when it occurs alone.

  d. *Neural Therapy*

The theory behind this intervention is that injury can disturb the body's flow of energy via dysfunction of the autonomic nervous system [ANS], and results in pain and other problems mediated through the ANS. Neural therapy involves injections of a local anesthetic [usually lidocaine or procaine] by using the ANS's pathways to the cells where there has been a disruption of normal function. Neural therapy is said to help normalize the body's ANS [electrical energy], and thus, cellular function.

  e. *Acupuncture*

Acupuncture is believed to reduce pain by rebalancing the body's flow of energy and nerve function.

  f. *Botox™ Injections*

A preparation of highly diluted botulinum toxin type A, is injected into muscles with chronic spasm. Initial trials of botox injections were with muscles exhibiting the TrPs of MPS. This treatment is presently in the early stages of research for fibromyalgia syndrome.

2. *Chiropractic*

It is claimed that manipulation of the spine lessens pain by realigning subluxations, enhancing nerve transmission, and improving muscle function.

3. *Physiotherapy, Massage Therapy*

These therapies attempt to increase function and range of motion of joints and muscles.

4. *Craniosacral Therapy, Reiki*

These specific subtle techniques are said to readjust the body's internal "energy."

5. *Transcutaneous Electrical Nerve Stimulation [TENS]*

Patients have variable responses to TENS for temporary relief of chronic pain.

6. *Synaptic Electronic Activation Technology [S.E.A. Tech®] (169)*

It is claimed that S.E.A. Tech may be effective for longer term pain relief and has resulted in improved sleep patterns and alleviation of fatigue. It is contraindicated in pregnancy and in the presence of pacemakers.

7. *EEG Neurofeedback*

EEG neurofeedback, via light and/or auditory stimulation, is claimed to improve all FMS parameters, and normalize brain wave patterns.

8. *Bright Light Therapy*

High intensity light [1,500 to 10,000 LUX] is said to help stabilize serotonin and melatonin levels in the brain as well as the circadian rhythm. Used for seasonal affective disorders [SAD], sleep and fatigue. When given in the morning, it was not effective in resetting the FMS biological clock.

9. *Magnetic Therapy*

Various devices that generate pulse magnetic fields are under investigation. The magnetic pulser MPG4 (170) has been approved by Health Canada as a class II medical device to improve tissue oxygenation, blood flow and healing, reduce edema as a result of injury and to relieve chronic pain from osteoarthritis and musculoskeletal injuries. Some patients use mattresses impregnated with magnets for sleep enhancement and pain reduction. There are no controlled studies in FMS.

10. *EMG Biofeedback*

Biofeedback provides patients with feedback, which may help them to gain some voluntary control over their pain. This is a proven performer in FMS.

11. *Cervical Collars or Belts*
    These devices may help alleviate fatigue and pain but may run the risk of muscle weakening from under utilization.
12. *Negative Ionizer*
    Exposure to atmospheric negative ions, such as being near large bodies of water or via a portable negative ionizer is claimed to improve cognitive functioning and mood.
13. *Aromatherapy*
    The aromas and scents of various plant-derived essential oils are believed by some to have different properties, including having an influence on the hypothalamus through the olfactory system. It is claimed that they reduce pain, and enhance energy and improve the general sense of well-being.

G. Supplements and Herbs

Many patients consume nutritional supplements and herbal preparations for their potential relief of symptoms. Most of these supplements have not undergone strict scientific trials and the scientific evidence that that does exist comes from studies in different areas of medicine, such as: heart disease, arthritis, etc. Some patients have found supplements and herbs helpful while others have not. Use the same therapeutic principles given at the beginning of the pharmaceutical section [F] for ascertaining their effectiveness.

While each individual has a unique biochemistry and unique needs for various nutrients, *those with chronic illnesses may require additional nutrients to support the repair process.*

The following is an overview of some of the supplements and herbal remedies commonly used by patient with FMS for their FMS symptoms. Most of the claims are unsubstantiated. Particularly, data applying to FMS therapy is lacking. [This is NOT an endorsement for any commercial product.]

Typical dosages are as indicated–it is important to check the labels for recommended dosage for a particular product. It has been argued that malabsorption may be a problem for some FMS patients, so higher dosages of nutrients may be required. Sublingual drops, and colloidal or chelated products are absorbed in different locations or may be easier to absorb.

1. *Vitamins and Minerals*

Vitamins are not nutrients from which energy is derived in the same way that proteins, fats, and carbohydrates provide nutrition. Vitamins are generally cofactors which aid the enzymes of the body make optimal use of nutrients. The recommended intake is based on estimated amounts needed to prevent overt symptoms of deficiency. It does not address optimum levels in chronic illness or amounts required to support healing. When practical, a balanced vitamin profile with levels of vitamins A, E, B-complex, and C can be helpful to ensure that proper supplementation. It is not proven that supplemental vitamin therapy is better than would result from eating a wholesome balanced diet. Use of megavitamin therapy is to be discouraged because some vitamins can be toxic in high levels. The principles and vitamin supplementation strategy of Travell and Simons (57) have been found to be useful.

Some of the following claims are said to be relevant for the FMS patient.

a. *Vitamin E* is an antioxidant said to stimulate the immune system and is claimed to combat chronic illness, to stabilize nerve membranes, and reduce fibrin.
b. *B-Complex* helps with energy enhancement and stress reduction.
c. *Vitamin C* is an antioxidant that stimulates the immune system and is important for combating any chronic illness.
d. *Beta Carotene*, a precursor to vitamin A, promotes a healthy immune system which is important in combating chronic illness. Note that high levels of fat-soluble vitamins such as vitamins A and E can cause toxicity that may be difficult to remedy. Since excess vitamin A can contribute to musculoskeletal pain (171), beta carotene, which can act as a non-toxic source of vitamin A, is recommended.
e. *Calcium and Magnesium Maleate* are involved in muscle and nerve action as well as interaction. Calcium is involved with hundreds of enzymatic reactions that are vital to health and recovery. Vitamin D must be present for the absorp-

tion of calcium. Too much calcium can be as hazardous to normal nerve and muscle function as too little.

Magnesium maleate may lessen fatigue and help prevent muscle cramps. Level of evidence [LE] II: ± results. Said to be effective for fatigue when taken with malic acid in an open-label follow-up of FMS (172,173).

Some studies suggest a general calcium and magnesium deficiency in FMS (174-176). Calcium and magnesium are usually taken in a 2:1 ratio but FMS patients may require extra magnesium.

f. *Zinc* enhances nerve and muscle functioning, collagen formation, and healing. A zinc deficiency [not demonstrated in FMS] would facilitate nociception and cause increased pain (174,173).

2. *Supplements*

a. *Essential Fatty Acids [EFA]* are essential for prostaglandin synthesis, cellular membrane integrity and help combat dry skin. In addition to eating fish of cold water origin, an EFA supplement is recommended, e.g.,

- *Salmon oil* promotes nerve impulse transmission and blood flow.
- *Evening Primrose oil* promotes improved blood flow and neural function.

b. *Lecithin* is involved in muscle, nerve and brain function, and circulation.

c. *NADH* is felt to enhance energy and improve immune function.

d. *MSM [Methylsulfonylmethane]* promotes strengthening of connective tissue, and reducing joint pain.

e. *Glucosamine Sulphate* may promote mobility of joints and pain reduction.

f. *Glutamine* may improve growth hormone production and muscle functioning.

g. *Procyanidolic Oligomers [PCO], e.g., Grape Seed Extract*, and Pine Bark Extract are used for protection of muscles, and to prevent bursitis and arthritis.

3. *Herbal Remedies*

a. *Ginkgo Biloba* may improve cerebral blood flow and cognition.

b. *Siberian Ginseng* may help heal soft tissue damage and boost the immune system. Siberian ginseng is not a true ginseng and is substantially different from and gentler than ginseng panax. Siberian ginseng can be taken by both females and males.

c. *Valerian* is thought to improve sleep, and promote calmness and relaxation.

d. *Devil's Claw* may reduce joint pain.

e. *Cat's Claw* may reduce pain.

To get an accurate knowledge of any disease it is necessary to study a large series of cases and to go into all the particulars–the conditions under which it is met, the subjects specially liable, the various symptoms, the pathological changes, the effects of drugs . . . in the faculty of observation, the old Greeks were our masters, and we must return to their methods if progress [is] to be made.

*. . . Sir William Osler
Counsel and Ideals*

FIBROMYALGIA SYNDROME "PATHOGENESIS"

Findings of physiological and biochemical abnormalities (177-179) provide compelling evidence that clearly identifies FMS as a biological and distinct clinical disorder (180,181) involving many body systems. The following discussion examines the categories of involvement as if they were independent entities although it is unlikely for them to occur alone. As the interactions between the abnormalities within these diverse systems are better understood, it will be increasingly possible to integrate the pathogenesis of FMS into a model or several distinct models of a disease process. The principal goal of this section is to briefly summarize the clinical and laboratory abnormalities that distinguish FMS from healthy normal controls [HNC], from persons with other pain disorders, and from primary psychiatric or mood disorders.

A. Etiology

Most patients enjoyed a healthy active lifestyle prior to the onset of FMS. There is no known single initiating cause [etiology] however, genetics appear to play a factor in some patients while numerous physical events such as trauma, surgery, repetitive strain, childbirth, viral infections, and chemical exposure can be associated with the onset of FMS in other patients. Extreme or chronic stress may be risk factors but that has not been proven. In some cases there is no known prodromal event and the symptoms come on gradually.

Genetics: Biochemical markers provide a resource for the objective identification of FMS patients and suggest possible hereditary factors may contribute to the illness in some patients. In a survey of 124 FMS patients (182), 20 percent indicated that one first-degree relative had similar symptoms; and 2.4 percent indicated that at least two other family members were affected. However, relatives were not examined to confirm their symptoms were actually due to FMS. Yunus et al. (183) reported that in 40 families with at least two first-degree relatives, who met the ACR criteria for FMS (1), 74 percent of the siblings, 53 percent of the children, and 39 percent of the parents had FMS. While Buskila et al. (184) found an overall prevalence of 25 percent of first line relatives with FMS-like symptoms, it was 83 percent in mothers, 50 percent in sisters, 33 percent in daughters, 15 percent in sons and 0 percent in fathers. Affected and unaffected offspring did not differ with regard to anxiety, depression (183), global well-being, quality of life, and physical functioning, suggesting genetic rather than environmental involvement (184). Family members of FMS patients had lower pain thresholds than an ethnically matched sample from the general population (184). Data from these and other studies (185) suggest an autosomal dominant mode of vertical transmission inheritance (183,184). Preliminary results of measured human leukocyte antigens [HLA] suggest significant linkage to the HLA region in a subset of FMS patients, supporting a genetic basis for FMS with a linkage to the HLA region in that subset of patients (186).

An ongoing study of 160 nuclear families in which at least two family members have FMS, involves microsatelite scan of the entire genome (187-189). and selectively testing serum gene markers of hypothetical candidates. The findings to date suggest that at least two genetically different subgroups can be identified. One group, associated with a serotonin receptor gene is associated with early onset, mild pain severity, and low blood tryptophan. The other group, associated with a histocompatability locus antigen region gene is associated with a later onset of symptoms, more severe symptoms, and low blood serotonin levels. These findings clearly implicate genetics in defining the character of the FMS for a given individual.

Physical trauma: There is strong consistency in documentation that physical trauma such as a fall or motor vehicle accident, particularly a whiplash or spinal injury, can trigger FMS in some patients (190-198). In a study of 973 FMS patients (26), 19 percent attributed the onset of their symptoms to antecedent trauma. Greenfield et al. (190) reported that 23 percent of 127 patients developed FMS reactive to a physical trauma. A long-term follow-up study (199) of 176 post-traumatic FMS patients indicated that prodromal trauma was a motor vehicle accident for 60.7 percent, a work injury for 12.5 percent, surgery for 7.1 percent, sports-related injury for 5.4 percent and other traumatic events for 14.3 percent. When the body is exposed to excessive force, it affects the spinal column. A study conducted in Israel (195) showed that previously health people who suffered a whiplash injury in an automobile accident were much more likely [21.6 percent of 102 neck injury patients] to develop FMS compared to 1.7 percent of the control patients with lower extremity bone fractures. None of these patients had a chronic pain syndrome prior to the trauma. In another study (200), 40 percent of patients reported a neck injury and 31 percent reported a lower back injury as the precipitating injury prior to the onset of FMS symptoms. In whiplash patients, occult injuries may occur to the vertebrae and temporomandibular joints (201), and/or functional lesions in the neurological pathways (202). These injuries can result in distortion of sensory information from the muscular and articular proprioceptive system at a central level. Evaluation of the spinal canal diameter of 48 consecutive patients with whiplash injuries following a motor vehicle accident, revealed the cervical spinal canal was significantly smaller in patients with persistent symptoms than those who were asymptomatic, with the cervical canal being narrower in women (203). An acute injury, such as a cervical flexion/extension injury, may result in cervical cord compression in the presence of cervical stenosis with structural changes (204). and spinal cord dysfunction (205,206). Some FMS patients may have cervical myelopathy on the basis of spinal cord or cervicomedullary compression (205). Whiplash injuries and back sprain can overstretch or fray ligaments, which are difficult to heal, and can cause muscles to become taut and shorten (21). These studies, as well as the presentation of plausible etiological mechanisms (207), make a compelling argument that trauma does, in fact, play an etiological role in the development of FMS in some, but not all patients.

Psychological: The all too common assertion that FMS symptoms are the manifestation of underlying depression or other psychological difficulties is not supported by available data.

Depression: An early study of depression in FMS (208) reported that depression was more common in people who had FMS than in patients with rheumatoid arthritis [RA]. This finding was interpreted by many as showing that FMS was more likely to be caused by depression than was RA. A critique of this study was that interviewers who administered and interpreted the psychological tests were not blinded to the diagnosis of those being interviewed and may have been biased towards a psychological explanation for FMS while considering RA to be an inflammatory disorder. A later study (209), designed to blind the interviewer to the diagnosis of FMS or RA, by wrapping all but the face of each patient in a sheet to prevent disclosure of RA-deformed joints, disclosed that the frequencies of depression in RA and FMS were approximately the same at 30-40 percent. Kirmayer et al. (210) reported a 20 percent rate of depression in FMS. It is reasonable to conclude that the depression seen in a subset of FMS patients is more likely secondary, reactive depression and not the cause of the painful syndrome (211-213).

Effects of depressive symptoms: Another view has been that the pain and fatigue of FMS might be inappropriately amplified by the presence of depression or anxiety. A study described by Ward (214). evaluated the roles of mood or depression in modifying the perception of painful stimuli administered to RA patients. Depression, as measured by the self-administered Center of Epidemiologic Studies Depression instrument, explained less than 1.0 percent of the changes in pain and global arthritis status, so it was concluded that depression was an unlikely cause for the pain of RA. It seems reasonable to extrapolate that conclusion to patients with FMS. It is likely that depression in both conditions is reactive as a consequence of daily chronic pain, insomnia, physical limitation, compromised quality of life, and demotion from the person's status as an equal competitor in the arena of life to that of a person with an incurable illness.

Pathogenetic differences of FMS and depression: Patients with post-traumatic stress disorder and major depression tend to have hyperactivity of the hypothalamic-pituitary-adrenal [HPA] axis (215), which is resistant to dexamethasone suppression, while there is hypoactivity of the HPA axis in FMS patients (177,216-218). The levels of cerebrospinal fluid [CSF] substance P are substantially higher in FMS than in major depression (219,220). Pain is not a common feature of depression but even when depressed patients complain of pain they are not expected to exhibit the multiple, painful tender points so characteristic of FMS. Irritable bowel syndrome, bladder dysfunction, a history of unsuccessful carpal tunnel surgery, headaches, atopy, premenstrual syndrome, and endometriosis, which are commonly seen in FMS (221,222), are not especially common in depression.

Childhood abuse: Several attempts to implicate childhood or adolescent sexual or physical abuse in the etiology of FMS (223,224) have encouraged this view held by some health care providers despite repeated studies that have failed to find evidence in its support. For example, a retrospective study (225) compared anonymous responses of healthy normal controls with equal numbers of demographically comparable persons with FMS or RA. Approximately 40 percent of all study subjects experienced at least one stressful trauma before the age of 18 years but the differences between the groups were not statistically significant. This study also explored the role of confiding the traumatic events to a trusted person based on the hypothesis that as children, FMS patients might have internalized more than other groups. Both FMS and RA patients were actually more likely than the normal controls to have confided their problems to a trusted individual. In an editorial on the subject, Hudson and Pope (226) concluded that the evidence was just not there to implicate childhood sexual abuse in the etiology or pathogenesis of FMS.

Raphael and colleague conducted a definitive prospective study (227) involving adults [N+676] who, as children, were so severely abused that they were identifiable 20 years later from public court records. Neither the abused subjects nor the control group [N = 520] knew the objective of the study and the interviewers were blinded to the group designation. None of the abused groups differed significantly from the control group with regard to painful symptoms, painful illness, or unexplained pain. When lifetime major depressive disorder was examined as a factor in the symptoms reported by the study subjects, there was a relationship between unexplained pain and depression among those who had not been abused but no relationship among those with a history of physical abuse. This ingenious prospective study has negated most of the speculation relating FMS symptoms to sexual abuse. The same study showed that self-reported victimization was retrospectively perceived by patients to be related to their symptoms indicating that retrospective reporting can be misleading when a clinically devastating condition like FMS is driving the introspection.

Somatoform disorders: According to the DSM IV, Somatization Disorder must include four pain symptoms, two gastrointestional symptoms, one sexual symptom, and one pseudoneurological symptom, which cannot be explained by a general medical disorder. In addition, patients with Somatization Disorder usually have a long history of complaints beginning before age 30 whereas FMS generally has a discrete and often sudden onset and most commonly occurs between the ages of 35 and 50. The other somatoform disorders of

Conversion Disorder, Pain Disorder, Hypochondriasis, Body Dysmorphic Disorder, and Undifferentiated Somatoform Disorder, also must be clearly unrelated to a general medical condition, or be the direct effects of substance abuse. The medical model of FMS shows numerous physiological abnormalities, which points to dysregulated pain physiology including CSF levels of substance P, abnormal cortisol levels, and those demonstrated by brain SPECT scans, etc. Somatization can only be diagnosed by excluding general medical conditions. The FMS and somatization disorders cannot both be diagnosed to explain the same set of symptoms in the same patient.

B. Insomnia

The early studies by Moldofsky and Smythe (5,6) established that over 70 percent of FMS patients were aware that they slept poorly and awoke in the morning feeling unrefreshed. Many of those who were unaware of trouble with their sleep had abnormal findings upon objective testing. The typical clinical complaint has been that they go to sleep without much difficulty but then awaken one to three hours later with nocturnal vigilance, having great difficulty returning to sleep. Attempts to exactly reproduce these findings have met with limited success.

Laboratory sleep studies: The characteristic findings from polysomnographic electroencephalography [EEG] recordings have been dysfunctional sleep with inadequate time spent in the deep restorative slow wave [delta wave, stages 3 and 4 non-rapid eye movement [non-REM]] sleep and contamination of the remaining delta wave deep sleep with arousal wave patterns [rapid, alpha waves, 7.5-11 Hz] (228, 229). Evidence suggests a distinct relationship between poor sleep quality and pain intensity (230). A diminished 24-hour heart rate variability consistent with an exaggerated sympathetic modulation of the sinus mode may help explain sleep disturbances in FMS patients (231).

Other sleep disorders: Another source of confusion about FMS insomnia is that it is difficult to distinguish from other related sleep disorders (232-234), which can overlap with FMS. For example, people with *myofascial*

pain syndrome [MPS] often exhibit disturbed sleep (235,236) and many awaken with jaw pain, headaches, and a sense of unrefreshing sleep. In *sleep apnea*, the sleeper ceases to breathe for a prolonged period of time. In the *obstructive form* of sleep apnea, adipose tissue in the upper airway or a patulous tongue obstructs the upper airway during sleep, while in the *central form* [idiopathic, Undine's curse], the brain fails to trigger the autonomic nervous system to rhythmically contract the diaphragm during sleep. Approximately 40 percent of male FMS patients suffer from sleep apnea (112). *Nocturnal myoclonus* or the restless leg syndrome is characterized by rhythmic jerking of the legs during sleep, which interferes with restful sleep (237,238). One study (30) reported approximately a 50 percent rate of nocturnal myoclonus in FMS patients while another study reported a statistical significant 31 percent rate of nocturnal myoclonus in 137 FMS patients compared to 2 percent of controls (24). Evidence suggesting that nocturnal myoclonus may be related to an autonomic dysfunction of the sympathetic nervous system has intriguing implications for further study in FMS (237).

C. Neurocognitive Dysfunction

Cognitive deficits: It is apparent that a major site of disturbance in FMS is the brain but the pathogenesis of the cognitive problems is unclear. Considering the sleep loss and chronic headache associated with FMS, it not surprising patients complain of significant changes in their cognitive functions. They have difficulty remembering events, patterns of behavior, task-related protocols, and numbers, all of which had been second nature to them prior to the onset of FMS (239-243). One study suggests that it is not an impairment in accuracy but rather slower speed in information processing, possibly due to chronic pain, non-restorative sleep symptoms and mental fatigue, that affects the cognitive performance of FMS patients (242). The role of distraction [such as noise, non-sense conversation, or a requirement to multitask] in bringing out, or exacerbating, the cognitive defects of FMS is being recognized as critical to the demonstration of a defect.

Memory: The prefrontal cortex [PFC] helps to regulate the hippocampus in new memory production. It has been proposed that dysfunction of the PFC could impair the function of the hippocampus. The cognitive context of memories may be lacking or unavailable for integration; therefore, repetitive situations may be erroneously interpreted as novel (244).

Hypoactivity of the frontal lobes in the awake state may impair ability to focus on tasks (245). Dysfunction of the reticular formation in the brainstem may cause insomnia, which prevents the replenishing of neuronal glycogen stores used during waking hours (246).

Neurophysiologically, an increase in glutamate production that occurs when nitric oxide diffuses into the presynaptic region of nerve fibers, will strengthen the synaptic connections that are necessary for new memory production (244). Repetitive hippocampal neural firing during slow wave sleep strengthens short-term memory. REM sleep is also vital for consolidating new memories. Both these sleep states are dysfunctional in FMS patients (247, 242), leading to attentional dysfunction, difficulty in concentrating, and ease of distraction. The result can be poor initial learning and impaired memory production similar to that of myalgic encephalomyelitis/chronic fatigue syndrome [ME/CFS] (248).

D. Neurosensory Dysfunction

Mismanagement of sensory information: Research and clinical experience suggest there is a lower tolerance to noxious stimuli such as exposure to excessive noise, light, fast-paced and/or confusing environments. A significantly hypersensitive response to these auditory, visual and somatosensory stimuli may be a major factor in the production of some symptoms (249,250). Due to neurotransmitter/receptor dysfunctions, sensory information is not managed properly in the brain (251). *Gating* is the process whereby the prefrontal cortex [PFC] assigns relative importance to the sensory information it receives. Goldstein (251) has speculated that conditions like FMS and ME/CFS may suffer from the effects of abnormal gating due to dysregulation of the signal to noise ratio [for example–high relevance is given to insignificant distractions] resulting in patients being unable to exclude background noise. This dysregulation could be associated with overwhelming fatigue. A similar dysregulation also amplifies the sensory input of the olfactory system when previously tolerated foods, drugs and odors make one sick or give rise to panic attacks. This subset of FMS patients [about half] may also meet the criteria for multiple chemical sensitivity based on subjective questioning (252).

Mismanagement of motor information: It has been speculated that disruption in the planning phases for motor activities may result in clumsiness of actions such as difficulty in tandem gait, balance problems, weakness and ataxia. If FMS patients have a concomitant myofascial pain syndrome with trigger points in the sternocleidomastoid and masseter muscles [which are thought to influence proprioceptive input into the vestibular system], the result could be postural imbalances and dizziness (57).

E. Fatigue

The fatigue of FMS may be described as overwhelming tiredness, as muscle exhaustion, or as weakness but it is typically less intrusive or physically pervasive than in the ME/CFS (253-257). Electrode stimulation of the medial temporal lobe may cause sudden, severe fatigue (251) so it is tempting to speculate that a dysfunction in that brain region may be responsible for the spontaneous symptoms in affected individuals.

The failure of FMS patients to exhibit the normal attenuation of the sympathetic: parasympathetic ratio on heart rate variability of the cardiac sinus node at night may help explain morning fatigue in FMS patients (231).

F. Stiffness

Morning stiffness is poorly understood in all of the clinical settings (258-260). As FMS patients often exhibit many hours of morning stiffness despite apparent lack of evidence for inflammation, it may be relevant to comparatively study the physiology of morning stiffness in RA patients as they also exhibit a long duration [one or more hours] of morning stiffness [while the relatively less inflammatory arthritic disorders such as osteoarthritis [OA]

usually exhibit 5-15 minutes of morning stiffness]. Despite its elusive nature, morning stiffness is considered to be very important in diagnosing RA (260,261). and a preliminary criteria for clinical remission is reduced duration of less than 15 minutes (262).

Hazes et al. (259) reported a comprehensive assessment of morning stiffness in RA, which provided a model for its evaluation. Morning stiffness is more severe when RA is quite active and the terms "stiffness," "pain," and "limited movement" seem to have been used interchangeably as descriptors, but only a single word descriptor tended to be used during periods of remission or near remission. As with FMS patients, nearly all patients with RA had to change their morning routines and needed more preparation time to accommodate the stiffness. Vigorous physical activity the day before tended to increase the likelihood of morning stiffness. The authors took exception to the use of the term "morning" stiffness as about half of the patients also experienced a similar form of stiffness later on during the day, which usually occurred in association with a period of immobility [referred to as gelling phenomenon].

One attempt at identifying a marker disclosed a correlation of morning stiffness with changes in morning serum levels of hyaluronic acid [HA] among the RA patients (263). Similar correlations were seen with fucosylated serum haptoglobin in RA (264), and with red blood cell saturated fatty acids [r = 0.434] in psoriatic arthritis (265). It is of interest, in this regard, that serum HA was found to be dramatically elevated in FMS patients, even higher than in comparison patients with RA (266).

In animal models, serum HA was found to increase with inflammation and to correlate with the severity of the synovitis. Engström-Laurent and Hällgren (263) reported the resting morning serum HA level [before getting out of bed, 124 ± 104 mcg/L] was higher in RA patients than that observed [26 ± 9 mcg/L] with demographically matched healthy normal controls [HNC]. The elevated resting value of HA in RA correlated with the ESR [$r = 0.53$, $P < 0.01$] and serum haptoglobin [$r = 0.69$, $P < 0.001$] but did not correlate with the severity or duration of the morning stiffness. Others

(267,268) also found a lack of correlation of morning stiffness with a single measurement of serum HA in RA patients. However, when a second blood sample was drawn an hour after rising a significant increase [P < 0.001] in the serum HA level [RA 278 mcg/L versus NC 28 mcg/L] was disclosed (263). The change in serum HA above the resting level [delta HA] correlated with the duration of morning stiffness [P = 0.01]. By noontime on the same day, the increased HA level had fallen back to resting levels. These authors proposed that the sensation of morning stiffness may relate to plugging of capillaries or lymphatics by the degraded fragments of the high molecular weight HA, but that has not yet been confirmed. An unanswered question is whether the mechanisms for the stiffness in FMS are similar to those of RA despite the obvious differences in the extent of inflammation and the mechanical injury to joints in RA.

Muscle co-activation: This dysfunction could be a cause of weakness and stiffness. [see Skeletal Muscle Dysfunction]

G. Skeletal Muscle Dysfunction

Many FMS patients perceive deep muscle or even bone pain. Some of the FMS tender points [TePs] are located over muscle masses [lateral border of the trapezius, supraspinatus, lateral epicondyle, upper gluteal, and medial knee]. Adding these observations to the perception of fatigue and exercise-induced pain in FMS logically led to the concept that there may be some form of anatomic abnormality or at least an energy deficit in the skeletal muscles of people with FMS (269-271).

Simms (272) argued that the abnormal findings in FMS skeletal muscle disclosed (273). by nuclear magnetic resonance spectroscopy [^{31}P-NMR] and other methods of study were due to chronic deconditioning. The failure to identify any histologic or electron microscopic abnormality specific for FMS when contrasted to muscle tissue from controls (274), provided further support to the search for central nociceptive mechanisms.

Newer technology may still contribute substantially to our understanding regarding the role of muscle disease in FMS. Positron emission tomography [PET], ligand = 18F-Fluoro-deoxyglucose was used (275) to get more information on the metabolic rate of glucose utilization by a skeletal muscle in the lumbar region of two healthy volunteers and six female patients with FMS. Since a steady state is crucial to this process, the investigators used a hyperinsulinemic euglycemic insulin clamp technique to stimulate the myogenic glucose uptake under stable plasma-glucose levels. The local metabolic rates of glucose utilization were estimated with a non-linear least squares fit on the three-compartment 18F-FDG-model. Under glucose clamp conditions patients with FMS showed a significantly [P < 0.001] lower metabolic rate of glucose [4.3 ± 21.1] mumol/100 g tissue/min compared with normal volunteers [8.5 ± 22.3 mumol/100 g/min]. Due to a significantly [P < 0.005] increased glucose backflow from tissue into the vascular space [k2 in the kinetic model], the rate of phosphorylation was markedly reduced in patients with FMS.

Myofascial pain syndrome: Another potential explanation for muscle pain in FMS is a recognized overlap with the myofascial pain syndrome [MPS], which is characterized by the presence of trigger points [TrPs] (57,58, 276). In FMS, there are multiple, symmetric tender points [TePs] which hurt locally when pressed, but do not refer pain. By contrast, a TrP reflects a regional phenomenon; it may be tender like a TeP, but also refers pain to a symptomatic zone of reference which is usually more distal. TrPs are not a diagnostic component of FMS but there is evidence to suggest that some FMS patients exhibit TrPs in addition to a full complement of 11 to 18 TeP (277). At least one trigger point was found in 68 percent of FMS patients and in 20 percent of the normal controls (277).

If a typical TrP is present in a FMS patient, a concomitant diagnosis of MPS should be made. The two conditions should be treated separately with the knowledge that TrPs in the setting of FMS are more resistant to treatment than when they present alone (278). The distinction between MPS and FMS is important to diagnostic classification, understanding of pathogenesis, clinical management, and outcome assessment. The MPS can probably be cured with aggressive therapy even in a FMS patient while there is no documented cure for

FMS. The pain of MPS is probably amplified when it occurs in the setting of FMS.

Muscle co-activation: It has been suggested (279,280) that a sense of muscle stiffness may occur when agonist and antagonist muscles are being co-activated at the same time by centrally mediated mechanisms.

Post-exertional malaise: Patients typically exhibit post-exertional fatigue and a sense of weakness with an increase in body pain and stiffness. For this reason, patients are often hesitant to exert themselves to avoid the consequences (281). It may take an inordinate amount of time for patients to regain the premorbid levels of physical function, mechanical competence, and confidence in their own abilities.

It has been demonstrated (282) that isokinetic muscle function [muscle contraction with movement of the joint] is more affected in FMS than is isometric function [muscle contraction against a joint that is not in motion]. A study using transcutaneous superimposed electrical impulses to test the degree of sub-maximal muscular contraction concluded there must be a major central nervous system component explaining the reduced muscular strength (283).

Muscle microtrauma: Bennett and colleagues believe that muscle microtrauma may play a role in the post-exercise exacerbation of pain in FMS through release of calcium ions (284, 52). When healthy muscles contract, nerve impulses [excitation coupling] activate a two-fold increase of calcium to release from the sarcoplasmic reticulum, which results in normal muscle contraction. However, if a muscle injury has caused the outside membranes of sarcomere to become leaky, calcium might be expected to pour in from the outside causing a non-physiological contraction on the injured sarcomeres. The elevated calcium ions in the muscles activate calcium dependent enzymes and could eventually lead to focal muscle necrosis and the development of fibrous tissue. This hypothesis has been developed in sports exercise literature (52,285-290), but the phenomena have not been demonstrated in patients with FMS. However, based on this hypothesis, it is recommended that FMS patients avoid eccentric power exercises and build up their strength gradually to avoid further muscle injury (52,290).

H. Sensory Processing

Healthy normal individuals generally do not perceive a four kilogram digital pressure stimulus as being painful. By contrast, that amount of pressure, or even substantially less causes a deep aching pain at multiple anatomically defined tender points on the bodies of people with FMS (1). This finding in FMS represents a lower-than-normal pain threshold and meets the clinical definition of a neurophysiologic phenomenon called "allodynia" (291). Allodynia is defined as a lower than normal pain threshold or a perception of pain resulting from a stimulus which would not be painful for a normal individual (291). This definition distinguishes allodynia from the term hyperalgesia, which refers to an overly aggressive response to a stimulus that is known to be painful and expected to cause pain. For that reason it was proposed (292). that FMS could be described as "chronic, widespread allodynia."

There were at least two implications from such a view. Firstly, FMS appears to represent a very unique opportunity to better understand the process of disordered nociception. Secondly, neurochemicals, which had earlier been shown to induce or influence allodynia in animals, should be studied in FMS. To act upon these concepts, effective clinical tools, including valid measures of pain severity have to be developed.

The most prominent manifestation of FMS has been its nearly constant, widespread, burning, stabbing, aching, nagging or exhausting pain in soft tissues that can be exacerbated by non-noxious deep pressure (293). That typical pain pattern figured prominently in the development of sensitive and specific criteria for the clinical classification of FMS (1). It is, therefore, not surprising that FMS researchers have focused on the basic mechanisms of pain signal processing.

When pain is the symptom, the physiological process is called "nociception" (294). The normal process of nociception involves peripheral tissue injury which activates afferent, unmyelinated A-delta and C-fibers to release pro-nociceptive neurochemicals at synapses in lamina I, III, and V of the spinal cord dorsal horn. As these neurochemicals diffuse away from the surface of the afferent neuron within the synaptic cleft, they can have any one of three fates: binding to their designated receptor on the synaptic surface of the target spinal neuron, inactivation by enzymes residing within the synaptic cleft, or re-uptake salvage back into the afferent neuron that released it. If the magnitude of the chemical stimulus is sufficient, the wide dynamic range spinal neuron will depolarize and carry the message of pain across to the contralateral side of the cord and up toward the thalamic nucleus of the mid-brain via the spinothalamic tract. From there it is communicated to other mid-brain nuclei, to the sensory cortex and to the prefrontal cortex where it influences mood.

A comprehensive biological model of the important role of the central nervous system [CNS] and autonomic nervous system [ANS] in FMS is emerging, in which the normal coordination between the brain and the other body systems is disrupted in many ways.

I. Neurochemical Factors

Neurochemicals and neurotransmitters: The roles of neurochemicals as neurotransmitters in the process of nociception and allodynia have been studied extensively in animals (295). with findings at least theoretically relevant to human FMS (292). This line of reasoning has led to the measurement of neurotransmitter levels in biological fluids obtained from FMS patients. Two classes of biochemical participants in the nociceptive process which appear to be important to FMS are pro-nociceptive neurochemicals [exemplified by the neuropeptide, substance P and by the excitatory amino acid glutamine] and anti-nociceptive neurochemicals [exemplified by the biogenic amines, serotonin and norepinephrine]. One hypothesis for the pathogenesis of the pain reported by FMS patients is that it represents a chemical pain amplification and distortion of the normal nociceptive process. If the problem is pain amplification, the underlying mechanism could be too much pronociceptive activity or too little antinociceptive activity, or some combination of both.

Pronociceptive agents: These are chemical mediators that would tend to drive the process of nociception, if there was a noxious stimu-lus. Greater than normal concentrations of these agents would facilitate or amplify pain.

Substance P [SP]: It is an 11 amino acid neuropeptide, which has several important roles in the process of nociception. Activated, small, thinly myelinated A-delta and C-fiber afferent neurons release SP into laminae I and V [A-delta] and laminae II [C-fiber] of the spinal cord dorsal horn. With random interstitial diffusion, SP or its C-terminal peptide fragment makes contact with neurokinin-1 [NK1] effector receptors. The mechanism of SP action in the dorsal horn of the spinal cord is not entirely clear but it apparently facilitates nociception by "arming" or "alerting" spinal cord neurons to incoming nociceptive signals from the periphery. Of course, SP released by the afferent nerve fibers into the dorsal horn of the spinal cord can also diffuse out into the extracellular space and from there to the CSF where it can be measured as CSF SP.

Substance P can be manipulated to induce allodynia in animal models. German investigators (296) examined the effects of administering SP intrathecally to rats. They observed a SP dose-dependent increase in the number of peripheral nerves and/or fiber types that were effective in driving the dorsal horn neuron to relay a nociceptive message to the brain. Substance P caused an increase in the size or number of mechanosensitive receptive fields involving nociceptive neurons, and it induced a lowering of the threshold for postsynaptic potentials. All of these effects were consistent with the model, which views SP as a facilitator of nociception.

The concentration of substance P is normal in the saliva, the serum and the urine of people with FMS (297). Recent evidence (298) suggests, however, that SP levels correlate inversely with tryptophan [TRP] levels and 5HIAA levels in FMS serum.

Vaeroy et al. (299) were the first to recognize that the concentration of SP was elevated [approximately 3-fold] in the CSF of FMS patients compared with healthy normal controls [HNC] subjects. Their findings were reproduced in three other clinical studies (219,300, 301), with the average CSF SP level in FMS being two to three-fold higher than in the HNC.

In the second study of CSF SP in FMS patients, 87.5 percent of FMS exhibited CSF SP concentrations greater than the highest HNC value (219). Age and gender had no influence on the measured CSF SP levels but minor differences were related to ethnicity. A number of lumbar-level CSF samples was collected in three sequential numbered fractions. The CSF SP concentrations in these samples failed to define a cranial to caudal gradient of CSF SP concentration. Another experiment involved inducing noxious pressure on the lower body TePs, but there was no significant increase in the levels of CSF SP as might have been expected if the SP were coming primarily from local afferent dorsal horn neurons.

In each of the first four studies on CSF SP, the conclusions were based on only a single sample of CSF from each subject. To answer that question of whether the CSF levels of SP were stable or fluctuated with the patient's symptoms, 28 lumbar level CSF samples were collected from the same medication-free patients an average of 12 months after the first medication-free sample had been obtained (302). "Medication-free" means that for two weeks the FMS patients discontinued all medications believed to be helpful in treatment of FMS symptoms. There was, on average, a slight increase in the concentration of CSF SP over time, which correlated directly with a small clinical change in pain/tenderness occurring over the same period of time. These findings imply that CSF SP may be integrally related to changes in the severity of the symptomatic pain of FMS. It is of interest that the regional cerebral blood flow [rCBF] of the thalamus and caudate nucleus in FMS correlates inversely with the level of CSF SP (303).

An important question is whether elevated CSF SP is unique to FMS. An earlier report (304) indicated that SP was lower than normal in a variety of chronic, painful conditions like low back pain. Spinal fluid SP is lower than normal in idiopathic pain diseases and in chronic neurogenic pain syndromes including diabetic neuropathy. Finally, both CSF SP and CSF met-enkephalin were normal in chronic pain patients. Patients with pain from herniated discs had normal CSF SP but CSF SP was mildly elevated in patients with severely painful osteoarthritis of the hip and normalized in those subjects after most of the pain had been relieved by total hip arthroplasty (305).

Experience with spinal fluid neuropeptides in San Antonio now includes analysis of SP in CSF collected from over 300 clinical subjects (306). Among them have been over 150 primary FMS patients and more than 50 HNC. Disease control groups, included more than 30 subjects with FMS associated with another painful condition. A smaller group of 14 subjects had other painful conditions, but lacked FMS. Only the HNC CSF SP values were significantly different from those found in the primary FMS patients.

The FMS study group at the University of Alabama at Birmingham (301) has shown that the higher CSF SP levels in FMS correlated with a decrease in regional cerebral blood flow [rCBF] within the caudate nucleus and thalamus of the same FMS patients. The reason for this relationship is not yet clear. It is not likely that the high levels of SP caused the apparent vasoconstriction because SP is known to be a potent dilator of cerebral vessels, provided that the vascular endothelium of those vessels is intact. It is possible that neuropeptide Y (177) or dynorphin-A (307). could cause the decrease in blood flow since both are known to be potent vasoconstrictors and both are elevated in FMS. One could speculate that the excess SP is produced in response to tissue hypoxia, as an attempt on the part of the CNS to restore more normal blood flow. That explanation seems unlikely, however, because major brain hypoxic injury [ligation of an internal carotid artery in rats] causes a substantial decrease in brain tissue levels of SP. Of course, not being able to immediately explain a biological finding does not negate it. As with many past observations, this finding may need to hibernate for a while until the key to understanding it is disclosed by further research.

Nerve growth factor: An exciting recent development in the study of CSF SP in FMS was the finding of elevated levels of nerve growth factor [NGF] in the CSF of primary FMS patients, but not in FMS with an associated painful condition (308). This peptide neurotransmitter is believed to facilitate the growth of SP-containing neurons and to be involved in the process of neuroplasticity. For these reasons, NGF could be critical to the initiation or perpetuation of the painful symptoms of FMS. If so, the next task would be to learn why NGF would only be elevated in the CSF of people with "primary" FMS.

Calcitonin gene-related peptide [CGRP]: This neuropeptide is currently somewhat of a mystery because it co-localizes with SP in afferent neural pathways but the only function attributed to it is competitive inhibition of the peptidase enzymes which degrade SP. In patients with diabetic neuropathy, CSF CGRP correlated highly with the concentration of CGRP in the peripheral nerves undergoing ischemic injury. In FMS, CSF CGRP was found to be numerically but not significantly higher than in HNC CSF (309). Considering that, it was surprising that CGRP in FMS CSF correlated inversely with the pain threshold, directly with the number of tender points by dolorimetry, directly with depression, and indirectly with the CSF 5-hydroxyindoleacetic acid [5-HIAA] concentration. The inverse correlation with 5-HIAA ties the 5-hydroxytryptamine [5-HT] [serotonin] pathway to peptide mediators at the spinal cord level CSF. No such clinical correlations were found with CGRP in the normal control CSF.

Dynorphin A: Recent data from animal systems has led one author to hypothesis a very important role for CSF dynorphin A in FMS (179) that must be followed-up with a prospective study. When high concentrations of dynorphin A were administered intrathecally to rats, the animals developed a flaccid paralysis. Intermediate concentrations of dynorphin A were less damaging but caused a persistent allodynia (310). The mechanism responsible for these effects appeared to involve N-methyl-D-aspartate [NMDA] receptors rather than the expected kappa-opioid receptors. Increased production of dynorphin A has been known to occur in animal experiments in which the spinal cord was constricted or otherwise injured. Under those circumstances, administered antibodies to dynorphin A reduced the severity of the deficit resulting from such injury. On the other hand, when dynorphin A was allowed to induce spinal cord injury, the damage appeared to be irreversible.

Another puzzle that must be explained was the fact that SP and dynorphin A were both elevated in the same FMS CSF samples (307). Dynorphin A can inhibit the release of SP after an acute noxious stimulus. More information is needed on this subject.

Excitatory amino acids [EAAs]: There are a number of EAAs which are known to play a role in the nociceptive process (294,311-324). Some of them, such as glutamine and asparagine, are known to be pronociceptive. They are released by the afferent neuron and activate receptors known as N-methyl-D-aspartate [NMDA] receptors. Others are suspected of modulating rather than facilitating the process of nociception. An important role of the amino acid arginine is the production of nitric oxide with subsequent release of citrulline. The potential importance of these excitatory amino acids to the symptoms of FMS was highlighted by several studies (103,104,325) in which patients with FMS were treated with drugs that inhibited the activation of the NMDA receptors by the excitatory amino acids. The evidence suggests that ketamine, an NMDA inhibitor, is able to substantially reduce the severity of FMS pain in about one-third to one-half of FMS patients. It is thought that both magnesium and zinc may influence the NMDA receptors so magnesium and/or zinc deficiency could facilitate nociception and lead to greater pain (174,173).

A study of the concentrations of EAAs in the spinal fluid of FMS and HNC was conducted because EAAs also appear to transmit pain. It was hypothesized that CSF EAAs may be similarly involved in this syndrome. It was found that the mean concentrations of most amino acids in the CSF did not differ amongst groups of subjects with primary FMS [PFMS], FMS associated with other conditions [SFMS], other painful conditions not exhibiting FMS [OTHER] or age-matched, healthy normal controls [HNC]. However, in SFMS patients, individual measures of pain intensity, determined using an examination-based measure of pain intensity, the tender point index [TPI], covaried with their respective concentrations of glutamine and asparagine, metabolites of glutamate and aspartate, respectively. These findings suggested that re-uptake and biotransformation mask pain-related increases in EAAs. Individual concentrations of glycine and taurine also correlated with their respective TPI values in patients with PFMS. While taurine is affected by a variety of excitatory manipulations, glycine is an inhibitory transmitter as well as a positive modulator of the N-methyl-D-asparate [NMDA] receptor. In both PFMS and SFMS patients, TPI covaried with arginine, the precursor to nitric oxide [NO], whose concentrations, in turn, correlated with those of citrulline, a by-product of NO synthesis. These events predict involvement of NO, a potent signaling molecule thought to be involved in pain processing. Together these metabolic changes that covary with the intensity of pain in patients with FMS may reflect increased EAA release and a positive modulation of NMDA receptors by glycine, perhaps resulting in enhanced synthesis of NO.

Antinociceptive agents: These are chemical mediators that would tend to inhibit the process of nociception if there were a noxious stimulus. Lower than normal concentrations of these agents would tend to control or limit the severity of pain from a noxious stimulus.

N-Terminal fragment of substance P: The data from one study suggested that there might be a weak negative correlation between CSF SP levels and pain in FMS (219). That correlation is the opposite of the strong direct correlative relationship that was predicted. An intriguing hypothetical explanation was related to a proteolytic product of SP. Intact SP can be proteolytically cleaved by SP endopeptidase to produce two main peptide fragments, the C-terminal [SP_{5-11}] and the N-terminal [SP_{1-7}] (326). Intact SP and its C-terminal peptide bind to the NK_1 receptor to facilitate nociception. The N-terminal fragment of enzymatically cleaved SP activates another receptor to effect potent anti-nociception. As the measured concentration of SP increases, activation of the N-terminal receptor could progressively counteract the nociceptive effect of the C-terminal portion of SP on the NK_1 receptor (327,328). For example, the N-terminal fragment is known to decrease the numbers of NK_1 receptors on the surfaces of the spinal neurons.

Met-enkephalin-arg-phe: The concentration of met-enkephalin-arg-phe, which is supposed to exert an antinociceptive effect in the spinal cord, was found to be significantly decreased among a group of Swedish FMS patients when compared with HNC (300). This is the expected finding if one were to predict that an enkephalin deficiency would increase the magnitude of nociception.

Other endorphins: Other endogenous endorphins were considered as possible contributors to the pathogenesis of FMS (307). Neither CSF β-endorphin [mμ-opioid receptor] nor dynorphin A [kappa-opioid receptor] were low in FMS CSF. Actually, the surprise was that the concentration of dynorphin A in FMS CSF was elevated. That finding could indicate an attempt on the part of the endogenous opioid system to balance the increased nociception. Alternatively, it could have very different implications that could not have been predicted in 1991.

Serotonin: Animal studies have provided some fascinating clues regarding the function of 5HT in the mammalian central nervous system [CNS]. Dietary protein is digested in the gut and the resulting tryptophan is absorbed through the intestinal mucosae. It is carried by albumin to the blood brain barrier [BBB] where TRP is taken up by an energy-dependent process for delivery to the brain stem raphe nucleus. The raphe neurons oxidatively decarboxylate TRP to 5HT and package it for axonal delivery at synapses in brain and spinal cord locations. For example, 5HT is released by raphe axons into the caudate nucleus and within the dorsal horn region at all levels of the spinal cord. In the spinal cord, 5HT is known to inhibit the release of SP by afferent neurons responding to peripheral stimuli. In this regard, it is interesting to note that raphe neurons also contain SP in concentration inversely proportional to the 5HT concentration. The role of 5HT in the caudate nucleus is less clear but it most likely is involved in regulating the magnitude of the signal relayed on the cerebral cortex.

A surprising observation from a murine model is that increased SP in the brain increases 5HT levels in the spinal cord, which in-turn decreases release of SP into the spinal cord. Thus, there seems to be an inverse relationship between brain SP and spinal cord SP concentrations. If these observations are applicable to human FMS, one would expect low brain tissue levels of both 5HT and SP, while spinal cord 5HT concentrations would be low and spinal cord SP would be high.

Moldofsky and Warsh (329) were the first to suggest that 5HT might be involved in the pathogenesis of FMS, both in failing to attenuate persistent pain and to correct insomnia. They found a clinical correlate between FMS pain and the plasma concentration of TRP, which was supported by Yunus et al. (330). More recently, the serum and cerebrospinal fluid [CSF] of FMS patients were found to exhibit low concentrations of TRP (331,332). Early findings of a low serum concentration of 5HT were supported by other investigators (333,334). It is now apparent that the low serum 5HT in FMS is due to low levels of 5HT in their peripheral platelets (335).

The levels of 5HT have not yet been reported in FMS CSF but the levels of its immediate precursor 5-hydroxy-TRP and its metabolic product 5-hydroxyindole acetic acid have been. Both were found to exhibit lower than normal concentrations in FMS CSF relative to the CSF of HNC (332,336). In addition, 5HIAA was measured in the 24-hour samples of patients with FMS and compared with the results from HNC (178). The rate of 5HIAA excretion was significantly lower in FMS than in the HNC. These findings are only indirect evidence to suggest that something is really amiss body-wide with the production and/or metabolism of 5HT in FMS. Perhaps the most critical location for such a deficiency would be in the CNS.

A novel and rather appealing hypothetical explanation for both the low serum TRP and 5HT in people with FMS was proposed by Klein et al. (337). They reported finding high titers of antibodies [IgG, IgM, anti-5HT which cross-reacted with TRP] in the serum of FMS patients relative to normal controls and in controls with rheumatic conditions. Their data raised the possibility that an autoimmune process might be responsible for the low levels of 5HT in FMS sera and platelets. Subsequently, two groups in the U.S. have reexamined this question using solid-phase radioimmunoassays [RIAs] (338,339). Sought were IgG and IgM antibodies to 5HT and neurophysiologically important gangliosides [monosialo- and asialo-Gm1] that serve as effector receptors for 5HT. Sera were obtained from individuals in each of three clinical groups [FMS, RA, and HNC]. Both groups came to the same conclusion, that

serum antibodies to 5HT or to 5HT receptors were not increased in FMS.

The much higher prevalence of FMS among females than among males has led to speculation regarding gender-specific causes. For example, in an epidemiological study of a Mid-Western community (340), the curves representing pain thresholds [sensitivity to a pressure stimulus] in men and women consistently showed lower values for women. Since the examination component of the ACR criteria for FMS involves the response to a fixed pressure stimulus of 4 kg, it is not surprising that the ACR criteria have identified more women than men with FMS.

Understanding of the mechanisms responsible for this gender-related difference in pain thresholds is incomplete. Measurements of female hormones have not been very fruitful. A highly probable explanation for gender-related differences in pain perception has come from an unlikely source-positron emission tomography [PET] of the brain. A group of Canadian neuroradiologists (341) were studying the CNS synthesis and metabolism of 5HT. They administered a radionucleotide-tagged analog of tryptophan [5-methyl TRP] to healthy adults of both sexes and measured the rate of its conversion through methyl-5HT to methyl-5-hydroxyindole acetic acid [Me-5HIAA]. The ligand conversion rate was significantly lower [by about seven-fold] in women than in men, providing a logical basis for a gender-related differential in antinociceptive activity. In addition, depletion of endogenous, unlabeled TRP by administration of a TRP-depleted amino acid mixture resulted in a seven-fold drop in 5HT synthesis among males but an even more dramatic 42-fold decrease among the women. While the rate of serotonin synthesis in the brain is related to gender as are estrogen or androgen, it is not difficult to imagine that there may have been a divergence between the two gender related systems during embryological development. Other investigators have not confirmed the findings of these investigators, nor has the technology yet been applied to people with FMS. Nevertheless, the concept provides a model to explain the observed gender-related differences in pain sensitivity and potentially could explain why females might be at greater risk for developing chronic wide-spread allodynia in response to painful injury.

J. Effector Receptor Blockaid

Increasingly, it is becoming possible to stimulate [agonist] or to inhibit [antagonist] the action of specific neurochemical effector receptors. The effector receptors must be distinguished from the reuptake receptors such as those that are blocked by the selective serotonin receptor inhibitors. Examples of the effector receptors would be the neurokinin-1 [NK1] receptor for substance P (342,343). or the N-methyl-D-aspartate [NMDA] receptor for the excitatory amino acids (316,321,344-346). As new ligands for these receptors become available, it is likely that new information can be learned about FMS by agonist or antagonist effects.

The role of the NK1 receptor in FMS was examined (347) by oral administration of a compound, called CJ-11,974. It had previously exhibited high avidity for the NK1 receptor and inhibition of substance P effect in animal experiments using dosages that were achievable in humans. Outcome assessments included function, pain, sleep, and psychological measures. The findings were that the dysesthesia of the hands were significantly improved by this therapy and the severity of the depression was dramatically reduced but the overall subjective perception of pain and the pain threshold measures were not significantly affected. The agent was generally well tolerated by the patients but a few patients who developed liver function abnormalities that resolved after discontinuing the drug raised concern.

K. Neuroendocrine

Many of the symptoms of FMS overlap those observed in patients with hormone deficiencies. That observation has led to the study of neuroendocrine function in FMS (177,217, 284,348-354). Subsets of people with FMS exhibit functional abnormalities in the hypothalamic-pituitary-adrenal axis [HPA Axis] (177,217,348-352), in the sympathoadrenal system [Autonomic] (231,355-358), in the hypothalamic-pituitary-thyroid axis [HPT Axis]

(349,175), in the hypothalamic gonadal axis [HPG Axis] (175), and/or in the hypothalamic-pituitary-growth hormone axis [HPGH Axis] (284,353, 354).

Hypothalamic-pituitary-adrenal [HPA] axis: The adrenocorticotropin hormone [ACTH] response to administered corticotrophin releasing factor [CRF] or to insulin-induced hypoglycemia and exercise was abnormal in FMS (177,350,351). It appears that there may be diurnal rhythm abnormalities in cortisol production and that the epinephrine response to physiological stress may be blunted. The responsible mechanisms have not yet been clearly delineated but there is considerable evidence to suggest that this system is regulated in part by serotonin [via $5HT_1$ and/or $5HT_2$ receptors] (359-364), and by norepinephrine (365,366), so the demonstrated deficiency of these neurotransmitters in FMS (336) could have far reaching neuroendocrine effects. The HPA axis is also influenced by substance P, so the elevated levels of this neurotransmitter that have been documented in FMS (219,300,301) could contribute to the dysfunction of the HPA axis. Finally, interleukin-6 appears to play a role in the regulation of the HPA axis (367), so the generation of cytokines in people with FMS is under scrutiny (368-370).

Glucocorticoid treatment: In the light of the abnormal regulation of the HPA axis in FMS, it is perhaps surprising that administration of glucocorticosteroid medications to people with primary FMS does not improve their symptoms (371). Conversely, substantial improvement of FMS symptoms may result from otherwise indicated corticosteroid treatment of patients with RA or systemic lupus erythematosus [SLE].

Hypothalamic-pituitary-gonadal [HPG] axis: Among patients with FMS, there are abnormalities in the hypothalamic-gonadal axis (175,372), such as a lower response of lutenizing hormone and follicle stimulating hormone in response to a hypothalamic stimulus. There even seems to be a worsening of the FMS symptoms of premenopausal women in association with the menstrual phase of the monthly cycle (373,374) compared with the ovulatory phase. Postmenopausal women seem to be more symptomatic than premenopausal women (374).

Despite these findings, it is not clear that such abnormalities can explain the gender specificity of FMS. A more likely scenario is that a gender-specific difference in the regulation of biogenic amine production in the brain is responsible (341).

Sex hormone treatment: Based on apparent dysregulation of the HPG Axis and the perception that postmenopausal females are more symptomatic than their younger cohorts, it would be tempting to propose sex hormone replacement therapy [HRT] for people with FMS. Unfortunately, it is not yet clear that hormone replacement is a therapeutically effective intervention in postmenopausal females, nor are there enough males with demonstrated androgen deficiency to conclude that administration of androgens to males with FMS is useful. It is thought that such therapeutic decisions would be made on the same basis as if the patient did not have FMS.

Hypothalamic-pituitary-growth hormone [HPGH] axis: Growth hormone was studied because it was known to be produced during delta wave sleep which many FMS patients fail to achieve normally (5). Growth hormone is difficult to measure because its release is pulsatile and its plasma half life is short. An alternative means of monitoring growth hormone production has been to measure the plasma levels of insulin-like growth factor-1 [IGF1, previously somatomedin C], which has a long half-life. An age-adjusted deficiency of IGF1 has been documented in a large number of FMS patients relative to normal controls (284, 353,375).

Growth hormone treatment: It is of great interest that administration of growth hormone to people with FMS reduces many of the symptoms associated with this disorder (354). It appears that response to human growth hormone [HGH] takes time since the treated subjects did not exhibit significant improvement until about three months of continuous therapy. Withdrawal of the drug usually resulted in recurrence of the symptoms. The dosage must be carefully monitored by measuring the insulin-like growth hormone-1 [IGF1] levels to avoid the development of gigantism and other potentially serious side effects. Regular injection therapy with this hormone is not univer-

sally appealing to FMS patients although it is remarkable how well they adapted to its use in the research study. To date, the cost of such therapy is too expensive [approximately US $1,000.00/month] to allow its widespread clinical use despite the fact that a HGH and IGF1 deficiency is demonstrable and administration of HGH is effective against at least some of the FMS symptoms.

Hypothalamic-pituitary-thyroid [HPT] axis: It has been suggested that thyroid hormone deficiency might cause FMS or at least mimic some of the typical FMS symptoms (175, 376-379). The production of thyroid stimulating hormone [TSH] and thyroid hormone in response to hypothalamic thyrotropin-releasing hormone [TRH] has been studied (349,175). While the production of prolactin in response to TRH administration was significantly greater than normal, the same stimulus resulted in significantly deficient production of TSH, tetraiodothyronine [T4], and triiodothyronine [T3] compared with the responses of healthy normal controls.

Thyroid hormone treatment: Thyroid hormone levels should be checked in patients with a new diagnosis of FMS and periodically thereafter. Hormone replacement should be instituted if a deficiency is demonstrated. The preparation [T4 versus T3] to be administered is controversial. There is insufficient evidence to support the hypothesis that FMS is caused by abnormal thyroid hormone receptors or a deficiency of T3, like in the sick-euthyroid syndrome (380).

Calcitonin: In one study (175), the levels of total serum calcium and free serum calcium in FMS patients were both significantly lower than was found in a normal control group. This finding was associated with an unmeasurable level of calcitonin in the majority of the FMS patients. While the reason for this abnormality is not yet known, the low levels of calcitonin were secondary, attributed to the low calcium levels. Just why the parathormone [PTH] hormone levels were normal rather than elevated in these patients with what could have been symptomatic hypocalcemia is also unclear. In another study (176), hair calcium and magnesium levels were found to be significantly higher in FMS patients, suggesting a general calcium and magnesium deficiency.

Calcium and magnesium treatment: Hypocalcemia and hypomagnesemia have not been a recurring theme in the majority of studies where a complete chemistry panel is routinely obtained, so the finding of hypocalcemia by Neeck Riedel (175), and hypocalcemia and hypomagnesemia by Ng (176), need to be confirmed before they are considered to be a consistent finding in FMS. If calcium and magnesium deficiencies are demonstrated in a patient with FMS, they should be managed as it would be managed in a person without FMS.

L. Autonomic Nervous System

There is evidence to suggest that the autonomic nervous system is functioning abnormally in people with FMS (231,355-358,381). Patients with FMS exhibit orthostatic hypotension when tested with a tilt table. In this test, the subject is strapped to a table on hinges. Gradually, the table is raised until it is fully vertical and the subject's full weight is resting on the feet. In contrast to the situation when the patient is standing on the floor, the bracing on the table holds the legs straight and prevents the leg muscles from returning blood to the head. For a subject with autonomic neuropathy, blood and other body fluids will pool in the legs and the subject will become lightheaded or feel faint. At that point, the table is lowered and the symptoms resolve. In a study by Bou-Holaigah et al. (31), 12 of 20 [60 percent] of FMS patients who went 45 minutes at 70 degree tilt had a drop in systolic blood pressure compared to none of the controls. All 18 of 20 FMS patients who tolerated a 70 degree tilt for more than ten minutes had a worsening of widespread pain while the controls remained asymptomatic. Such abnormal autonomic control associated with sympathetic over activity has come to be called neurally mediated hypotension. Symptoms can include light-headedness while standing or rising from a recumbent position, cognitive difficulties, blurred vision, pallor, severe fatigue, tremulousness, and unexplained syncope. Rowe et al. (382) and Davis et al. (383) suggest that predisposing factors to NMH include low resting blood volume, excessive pooling of blood in the dependent vessels, and excessive loss of plasma volume during upright posture. It is not known why there is failure to effectively mobilize blood from the dependent splanchnic and limb vasculature, which decreases venous return and leads to an exaggerated sympathetic output (382). Further study needs to focus on the disturbances of the cerebral blood flow induced by orthostatic stress and whether NMH in FMS patients is secondary to a more generalized abnormality in the central nervous system.

The work of Martinez-Lavin and coworkers (231) has associated heart rate regulation abnormalities with the trouble FMS patients have getting deep, restful sleep at night. Electrocardiograms of FMS patients suggest their basal autonomic state has increased sympathetic and decreased parasympathetic tones (384). The value of their ratio decreases markedly during the night in healthy normal controls but fails to fall among the FMS patients in a manner parallel to the trouble they experience with achieving deep sleep. A 24 hour Holter monitor can be used to evaluate the normal regulation of the heart rate with respiration over time. The relative contribution of the sympathetic nervous system acceleration of the heart rate compared to parasympathetic nervous system as they affect heart rate variability provides an assessment of autonomic nervous system regulation of the heart rate.

Mineralocorticoid treatment: Some clinicians have found that administration of mineralocorticoids can reduce the severity of the neurally mediated hypotension, which occurs in some FMS patients (357). While that has been moderately successful in the management of some patients with ME/CFS, it is less clear that it is a useful treatment for people with FMS even when they are demonstrated to have a positive tilt test for autonomic dysfunction.

Morphological abnormalities of the red blood cells: FMS patients have exhibited marked morphological abnormalities in the red blood cells [RBC] population (385). These changes in the shape of the RBC tend to make them less flexible thereby impairing their ability to enter the capillary bed. The loss of flexibility may reduce the blood flow and thus the delivery rate of oxygen and metabolic nutrients into the tissue and also inhibit the ability to dispose of metabolic waste (386).

M. Central Nervous System Imaging

There has been a growing realization that many symptoms and signs of FMS originate from abnormalities of the central nervous system. For the purpose of this discussion, the central nervous system is composed of the spinal cord and the brain but not the peripheral nerves or the tissues that the peripheral nerves innervate.

Functional imaging studies: Functional imaging has become available to studies in FMS over the last ten years. Studies using techniques such as single photon emission computerized tomography [SPECT], positron emission tomography [PET], magnetic resonance imaging [MRI], functional magnetic resonance imaging [fMRI], and electroencephalographic spectral [EEG-S] assessment all provide support for the theory that there is altered processing of sensory input in FMS patients.

SPECT scan analysis has shown that regional cerebral blood flow [rCBF] in the thalamic, the caudate nuclei, and pontine tegmentum of the brain is low in FMS patients compared to healthy controls (387,388). Even more importantly, the magnitude of the effects seen in SPECT scanning of FMS patients correlates with their perception of pain (389).

Reduced thalamic blood flow in chronic pain states is further supported by a similar finding using PET scans in patients with unilateral chronic neuropathic pain (390), but there is a paucity of information about this methodology applied to the pathogenesis of FMS.

The use of EEG spectral assessment (391). for FMS patients has demonstrated dominance of slow wave delta activity, which can distinguish FMS from the myofascial pain syndrome [MPS]. The dominant slow wave delta activity allows for the specific diagnostic differentiation (392), and may prove to be a resource for alternative treatment (393). Analysis of the electrical characteristics of the signals of inappropriate muscle activity associated with tender points suggests a neurological origin (394, 395).

Preliminary MRI studies (205,206,396-398) of the brainstem and upper cervical spine have identified cervical stenosis in a subset of patients that met the criteria for FMS. Heffez et al. (27) noted that Chiari I malformation and cervical myelopathy due to spinal stenosis had been associated with symptoms similar to those found in FMS. Between 1998-2001, 270 patients with a diagnosis of FMS underwent clinical evaluation (27) by a neurologist and/or neurosurgeon as well as radiological evaluation by means of an MRI scan of the cervical spine and brain with special attention to the foramen magnum, along with a CT scan of the cervical spine in the neutral and extended position. This referred group was selective in that 59 percent of the patients reported antecedent craniospinal trauma within 3-6 months of the onset of symptoms, and it may have included more severe cases, [68 percent had left their job as a direct result of their illness]. Ninety-six percent of these patients had exertional fatigue, 95 percent had neck/back pain, 95 percent had fatigue, 92 percent had cognitive impairment, 88 percent had worsening symptoms with neck extension, 85 percent had instability of gait, 83 percent had subjective grip weakness, 80 percent had paresthesiae, 71 percent had dizziness and 69 percent had numbness of the hands/feet. On examination, 93 percent of patients showed a thoracic spinothalamic sensory level between T3-6, with hyperalgesia and allodynia to a cold or light pinprick stimulus. Sixty-four percent showed hyper-reflexia, and 57 percent showed recruitment, especially inversion of the radial periosteal reflex. A positive Romberg sign was observed in 28 percent, positive Hoffman sign in 26 percent, varying degrees of ankle clonus in 25 percent, impaired tandem walk in 23 percent, dysmetria in 15 percent and disdiadochokinesis in 13 percent. Neck extension and flexion caused an accentuation of pyramidal tract findings in 88 percent and 73 percent of the patients respectively, suggesting a mechanical etiology for the abnormal signs. In 20 percent of patients, a radiological diagnosis of Chiari I malformation could be made on the basis of tonsillar ectopia > 5mm in the mid-sagittal image. In 46 percent of patients, the anteroposterior [AP] mid-sagittal spinal canal diameter at the C 5-6 intervertebral disc space measured 10 mm or less with the neck placed in extension, a degree of stenosis consistent with symptomatic spinal cord compression. Other levels were also examined to diagnose cervical stenosis. Patients with abnormal neuroradiological findings consistent with compression of the cervical spinal cord or caudal brain stem were non randomly selected for surgically treated [N = 64] or nonsurgical [N = 44] treatment groups according to accepted clinical practice. These groups were virtually identical regarding sex ratio, mean age and duration of illness, history of craniospinal trauma, level of education and work history. The prevalence of symptoms and abnormal neurological findings did not differ between the 2 groups, nor did their quality of life, level of anxiety or depression [as measured by HADS and SF36 questionnaires]. At a 6-month follow-up there was a statistically significant improvement in the surgically treated group compared to the non-surgical group with respect to dizziness, limb numbness, pain, impaired balance and grip weakness. There was also improvement in symptoms of irritable bowel syndrome, impaired memory and concentration, and disorientation. A less significant improvement in headaches was noted, as well as non-significant improvements in fatigue, depression, insomnia, limb paresthesiae, clumsiness and cold intolerance. A significant improvement in quality of life score was noted. These outcomes [while they need to be extended and repeated by other groups], are encouraging. Evidence of cervical myelopathy during a careful routine neurological examination warrants neuroradiological examination of the brain and cervical spine and an appropriate neurological referral, since this study suggests a specific pathogenesis and treatment direction for a subset of FMS patients.

In a clinical observation in support of the brain tissue injury hypothesis of FMS [in personal communication from Rosner MJ], patients with central nervous system compressive neuropathy [brain stem-posterior fossa, e.g., Arnold Chiari malformation; or cervical cord-cervical spinal stenosis, whiplash injury] exhibited symptoms similar to those of FMS. In a recent study of FMS patients with Chiari I malformation, diagnosed by MRI (399), the levels of CSF SP were numerically higher than in the CSF of FMS patients who exhibited no such evidence of brain stem compression.

The use of fMRI for the study of FMS is still in its infancy. This technique involves conducting a continuous MRI examination of the brain while a variable is changed. Two preliminary studies to date have involved a pressure stimulus to the hand (400), or to the medial knee tender point on the right leg (401). Generally there have been three conditions: no stimulus, a painless stimulus, and a painful stimulus. The baseline noise in the MRI signal is subtracted from either the painless or the painful signal to give changes in activity related to the stimuli for various portions of the brain which are then overlaid on the static images of the MRI to establish the anatomic equivalents. The method clearly shows differences between FMS and controls with regard to the behavior of the brain to painless and painful stimuli. As with brain SPECT, there is consistent involvement of the thalamus and caudate nuclei, but in addition, activity is seen in the sensory cortex, the prefrontal cortex, occiput, and cerebellum.

A repetitive peripheral stimulation study (402) has tested the hypothesis that FMS patients might exhibit abnormal wind-up[2] at the level of the spinal cord dorsal horn. Wind-up was evoked both in controls and FMS subjects but there were clear differences by diagnosis group. The perceived magnitude of the sensory response to the first stimulus within a series was consistently greater for FMS subjects compared to controls, as was the amount of temporal summation within a series. Within a series of stimuli, FMS subjects reported increases in sensory magnitude to painful levels for interstimulus intervals of 2-5 seconds. By contrast, pain was seldom evoked at intervals greater than 2 seconds for control subjects. Following the last stimulus in a series, after-sensations were greater in magnitude, lasted longer and were more frequently painful in FMS subjects. These results have multiple implications for the general characterization of pain in FMS, for an understanding of the underlying pathophysiological basis, and for testing the efficacy of therapeutic interventions.

N. Respiratory System

Most patients with FMS experience chest wall discomfort and some have, at times, felt short of breath as illustrated in a brief case report (403). While no parenchymal abnormalities in the lungs have been demonstrated, there is convincing evidence for alveolar hypoventilation, probably secondary to chest wall pain (404), and for respiratory muscle dysfunction (405,406).

O. Gastrointestinal System

Irritable bowel-like symptoms of alternating constipation and diarrhea occur in approximately 40 percent of FMS patients (32,222, 256,407- 409). The mechanism for this association is unknown, but it is interesting to note that when a bolus of food is taken into the stomach, substance P and serotonin are normally secreted into the lumen and may have important effects on motility (410). Even less well understood is the relationship between FMS and inflammatory bowel disease, especially Crohn's disease reported in an Israeli study (411), but not found in a Norwegian study (412). The increased association of FMS with other inflammatory disorders such as systemic lupus erythematosus [SLE] (413,414), rheumatoid arthritis [RA] (17,415), and Sjogren's syndrome (414,416) is well recognized.

P. Urologic System

An association between interstitial cystitis and inflammatory bowel disease has been noted and the rationale discussed (417). A review (417,418) has summarized the evidence to suggest that there is also a relationship between interstitial cystitis and FMS. In a prospective study (419). designed to better understand this relationship, it was disclosed that patients with interstitial cystitis exhibited low peripheral pain thresholds [allodynia] like that of FMS.

FUTURE DIRECTIONS

Progress has been made in the knowledge and understanding of FMS but much more needs to be done. Future directions should emphasize the following components

A. Patient's Perspective

1. Support and validate the individual patient's suffering and limitations.

2. Assess patients honestly and treat them respectfully.
3. Provide up-to-date educational materials to patients and their meaningful others.
4. Provide hope for more effective interventions.
5. Establish an FMS patient registry.

B. Social Perspective of Society

Studies on impact of FMS on individuals and society should include:

1. An accurate estimate of the number of individuals with FMS, and their degree of disability.
2. An estimate of the economic impact of the condition on themselves, their families and society.
3. The social impact of FMS on interpersonal, community and national levels.
4. A plan to develop support structures and treatment strategies using the best scientific methods.

C. Caregivers

1. Encourage their participation in Continuing Medical Education [CME] programs to become knowledgeable about FMS and develop proper therapeutic and supportive relationships with people who have FMS.
2. Within the limits of their competence, encourage caregivers to cooperate in developing integrated treatment protocols.
3. Encourage caregivers to cooperate in research programs.

D. Research

It would be helpful if research studies distinguished between mild and severe cases, between newly diagnosed and those in chronic stages of FMS, and those with a comorbid diagnosis.

Further research is obviously needed on the pathophysiology of FMS. Targets should include:

1. The etiology of FMS including genetic components and prodomal events such as physical trauma.

2. The development of a deeper understanding of the role of the CNS in the genesis of symptoms.
3. Study of the role of injury to the CNS, in the development of independent pain.
4. Identify biological measures [laboratory tests and imaging markers] that distinguish FMS from healthy normal controls and disease controls.
5. Investigation of the influence of comorbid illnesses, such as myalgic encephalomyelitis/chronic fatigue syndrome and myofascial pain syndrome, on treatment protocol and/or prognosis.
6. Investigate which treatments are more beneficial in the acute stage and chronic stage of FMS.
7. Comparison of the performance of FMS patients with those with other musclo-skeletal disorders in the usual disability assessment tests and the impact of the symptoms on the patients' lifeworld. A major inclusion would be a comparison of the effect of the test on symptoms for a number of days following the test.

Clarification of this type of information in future studies will give a clearer picture as to whether the findings apply to most patients or only a particular subset of patients. It may be of assistance in determining what treatments or programs may be more appropriate for a particular patient subset. Although it is most important to keep in mind that each patient is unique and will require an individualized protocol, knowing results for different subsets of patients could make the search for effective remedies more rational and efficient.

Knowledge evolves, but in such a way that its possessors are never in sure of possession.

. . . Sir William Osler
The Evolution of Modern Medicine

NOTES

1. "Crashes" refer to a temporary period of immobilizing physical and/or mental fatigue.
2. Wind-up: continued firing up to a few minutes after the inputs cease.

REFERENCES

1. Wolfe F, Smythe HA, Yunus MB, Bennett RM, Bombardier C, Goldenberg DL, Tugwell P, Campbell SM, Abeles M, Clark P, Fam AG, Farber SJ, Fiechtner JJ, Franklin CM, Gatter RA, Hamaty D, Lessard J, Lichtbroun AS, Masi AT, McCain GA, Reynolds WJ, Romano TJ, Russell IJ, Sheon RP: The American College of Rheumatology 1990 Criteria for the Classification of Fibromyalgia: Report of the Multicenter Criteria Committee. *Arthritis Rheum* 33:160-172, 1990
2. Bennett R. [Chairman of expert panel], Kamper-Jorgenson F [Chairman of consensus panel]: The Copenhagen Declaration: consensus document on fibromyalgia. Myopain '92. *J Musculoske Pain* 1(3/4): 295-312, 1993.
3. Gowers WR: Lumbago: its lessons and analogues. *Br. Med J* 1:117-121, 1904.
4. Traut EF: Fibrositis. *J Am Geriatr Soc* 16:531-538, 1968.
5. Smythe HA, Moldofsky H: Two contributions to understanding the "fibrositis" syndrome. *Bull Rheum Dis* 28: 928-931, 1977.
6. Moldofsky H, Scarisbrick P, England R, Smythe H: Musculoskeletal symptoms and non-REM sleep disturbance in patients with "fibrositis syndrome" and healthy subjects. *Psychosom Med* 37(4):341-351, 1975.
7. White KP, Speehley M, Harth M, Ostbye T: The London fibromyalgia epidemiology study: the prevalence of fibromyalgia syndrome in London, Ontario. *J Rheumatol* 26(7):1570-1576, 1999.
8. Wolfe F, Ross K, Anderson J, Russell IJ, Hebert L: The prevalence and characteristics of fibromyalgia in the general population. *Arthritis Rheum* 38:19-28, 1995.
9. Croft P, Schollum J, Silman A: Population study of tender point counts and pain as evidence of fibromyalgia. *BMJ* 309:696-699, 1994.
10. Buskila D, Press J: Assessment of non-particular tenderness and prevalence of Fibromyalgia in children. *J Rheumatol* 20 (2):368-370, 1993.
11. Wolfe F, Anderson J, Harkness D, Bennett RM, Caro X, Goldenberg DL, Russell IJ, Yunus MB: Health status and disease severity in fibromyalgia: results of a six center longitudinal study. *Arthritis Rheum* 40:1571-1579, 1997.
12. Bennett R: The Scientific Basis for Understanding Pain in Fibromyalgia. *The Oregon Fibromyalgia Foundation http://www.myalgia.com*
13. Russell IJ: From clinical observation.
14. Wolfe F, Anderson J, Harkness D, Bennett RM, Caro X, Goldenberg DL, Russell IJ, Yunus MB: A prospective, longitudinal, multicenter study of service utilization and costs in fibromyalgia. *Arthritis Rheum* 40:1560-1570, 1997.
15. White KP, Speechley M, Harth M, Ostbye T: The London fibromyalgia epidemiology study: direct health care costs of fibromyalgia syndrome in London, Canada. *J Rheumatol* 26(4):885-889, 1999.
16. Mitchell DM, Spitz PW, Young DY, Bloch DA, McShane DJ, Fries JF: Survival prognosis in rheumatoid

arthritis: an eight year prospective study. *Ann Rheumatol Dis* 38:7-13, 1989.

17. Wolfe F: Non-articular symptoms of fibrositis, rheumatoid arthritis, osteoarthritis and arthralgia syndromes. *Arthritis Rheum* 25:S146, 1982.

18. Baker DG: Complications of rheumatoid arthritis. In: Rheumatoid Arthritis. An Illustrated Guide to Pathology, Diagnosis, and Management. Edited by HR Schumachernd EP Gall. *J.B. Lippincott*, Philadelphia, USA 15:1-18, 1988.

19. Erhardt CC, Mumford PA, Venables PJWW, Maini RN: Factors predicting a poor life prognosis in rheumatoid arthritis: an eight year prospective study. *Ann Rheum Dis* 48:7-13, 1989.

20. Kayfetz, D: Occipital-cervical [whiplash] injuries treated by prolotherapy. *Med Trail Tech Quart* 9-29, 1963.

21. Hauser RA, Hauser MA: Prolo Your Fibromyalgia Pain Away! *Beulah Land Press*, Oak Park, Illinois 2000.

22. Cathey MA, Wolfe F, Kleinheksel SM: Functional ability and work status in patients with fibromyalgia. *Arth Care Res* 1:85, 1988.

23. Yunus MB, Maise AT, Calabro IJ, Miller KA, Feigenbaum SL: Primary fibromyalgia [fibrositis] clinical study of 50 patients with matched normal controls. *Semin Arthritis Rheum* 11:151-171, 1981.

24. Yunus MB, Aldag JC: Restless legs syndrome and leg cramps in fibromyalgia syndrome: a controlled study. *Brit Med J* 312:1336-1339, 1996.

25. Russell IJ: Fibrositis/fibromyalgia [Chapter 23], in The Clinical and Scientific Basis of Myalgic Encephalomyelitis/Chronic Fatigue Syndrome. Editors: Hyde BM, Goldstein J, Levine P. *The Nightingale Research Foundation* 1992.

26. Lessard JA, Russell IJ: Fibrositis/fibromyalgia in private rheumatology practice: systematic analysis of a patient data base. 1989 [unpublished] Reported in: Russell IJ: Fibrositis/fibromyalgia [Chapter 23]. In: The Clinical and Scientific Basis of Myalgic Encephalomyelitis/Chronic Fatigue Syndrome. Editors: Hyde BM, Goldstein J, Levine P: *The Nightingale Research Foundation*, Ottawa, Canada, 1992.

27. Heffez DS, Ross RE, Shade-Zeldow Y, Kostas K, Shah S, Gottschalk R, Elias DA, Shepard A, Leurgans SE, Moore CG: Is cervical myelopathy overlooked in patients with fibromyalgia? Presented at the *European Section of the Cervical Spine Research Society*, Paris, France, June 12-15, 2002

28. DeJong RN: The Neurological Examination, 3rd edition. *Harcourt and Brace Publishers*, New York, NY 1967.

29. Leung F: Types of fatigue derived from clinical observation. Unpublished.

30. Romano TJ: Presence of nocturnal myoclonus in patients with fibromyalgia syndrome. *Amer J Pain Man* 9(3):85-89, 1999.

31. Bou-Holaigah I, Calkins H, Flynn JA, Tunin C, Chang HC, Kan JS, Rowe PC: Provocation of hypo-

tension and pain during upright tilt table testing in adults with fibromyalgia. *Clin Exper Rheumatol* 15:239-246, 1997.

32. Sivri A, Cindas A, Dincer F, Sivri B: Bowel dysfunction and irritable bowel syndrome in fibromyalgia patients. *Clin Rheumatol* 15:283-286, 1996.

33. Griep EN, Boersma JW, Lentjes EG, Prins AP, van der Korst JK, de Kloet ER. Function of the hypothalamic-pituitary-adrenal axis in patients with fibromyalgia and low back pain. *J Rheum* 25(7):1374-1378, 1998.

34. Janda V, Schmid HJA: Muscles as a pathogenic factor in back pain. *Int'l Fed of Orthopaedic Manual Therapists Proceedings*, New Zealand, 1980. In Janda Compendium, Vol 1. Distributed by *OPTP*, Minneapolis, MN, pg. 46.

35. Janda V: Muscles and cervicogenic pain syndromes. *Physical Therapy of Cervical and Thoracic Spine*. Edited by Grant R. Churchill Livingstone, New York, Edinburgh, London Melbourne, pg. 153-166, 1988. In: Janda Compendium, Vol. II. Distributed by *OPTP*, Minneapolis, MN, pg. 8.

36. Janda V: Muscles and motor control in low back pain: assessment and management. *Physical Therapy of the Low Back*. Edited by Twomey LT. Churchill Livingstone, New York, Edinburgh, London Melbourne, 253-278, 1987. In: Janda Compendium, Vol. II. Distributed by *OPTP*, Minneapolis, MN.

37. Seibel DG: Clinical musculoskeletal testing and examination of approximately 2,000 FMS patients. Mayfield Pain & Musculoskeletal Clinic, Edmonton, AB. Unpublished

38. Travell JG, Simons DG: Myofascial Pain and Dysfunction: The Trigger Point Manual: Volume 1: The Upper Extremities. First Edition. *Williams & Wilkins*, Baltimore, pg. 206-207, 1983.

39. Leung F: Supraclavicular swelling in fibromyalgia: possible sign of cord irritation. *J Rheum* 28 (suppl 63):21, July 2001.

40. Lewit K: Manipulative Therapy in Rehabilitation of the Locomotor System. Second Edition. *Butterworth Heinemann* 1991, pp. 1-345.

41. Maigne R: Diagnosis and Treatment of Pain of Vertebral Origin: A Manual Medicine Approach. *Williams & Wilkins, a Waverly Company*, Baltimore 1996.

42. Buchwald D, Garrity D: Comparison of patients with Chronic Fatigue Syndrome, Fibromyalgia, and multiple chemical sensitivities. *Arch Intern Med Sept* 154(18): 2049-2053, 1994.

43. Goldenberg DL, Simms RW, Geiger A, Komaroff AL: High frequency of fibromyalgia in patients with chronic fatigue seen in a primary care practice. *Arthritis Rheum* 33:381, 1990.

44. De Meirleir K, Bisbal C, Campine I, De Becker P, Salehzada T, Demettre E, Lebleu B: A 37 kDa 2-5A binding protein as a potential biochemical marker for chronic fatigue syndrome. *Amer J Med* 108(2):99-105, 2000.

45. Hendriksson D: Living with fibromyalgia: A study of the consequences for daily activities. [Doctoral thesis] Departments of Caring Sciences & Rheumatology, Linkoping University, Linkoping, Sweden.

46. Clark A: Being There: Putting Brain, Body and World Together Again. *Cambridge Mass, Bradford Books, MIT Press* 1997.

47. Karjalainen K, Malmivaara A, Van Tulder M, Roine R, Jauhiainen M, Hurri H, Koel B: Multidisciplinary rehabilitation for fibromyalgia and musculoskeletal pain working age adults. *Cochrane Database Syst Rev* 2:CD001984, 2000.

48. Burckhardt CS, Mannerkorpi K, Hedenberg L, Bjelle A: A randomized, controlled clinical trial of education and physical training for women with fibromyalgia. *J Rheumatol* 21(4):714-720, 1994.

49. Nicassio PM, Radojevic V, Weisman MH: A comparison of behavioral and educational interventions for fibromyalgia. *J Rhematol* 24(10):2000-2007, 1997.

50. Vlaeyen JW, Teeken-Gruben NJ, Goossens ME: Cognitive-educational treatment of fibromyalgia: a randomized clinical trial. I. Clinical effects. *J Rheumatol* 23(7):1237-1245, 1996.

51. Wigers SH, Stiles TC, Vogel PA: Effects of aerobic exercise versus stress management in fibromyalgia. A 4.5 year prospective study. *Scan J Rheumatol* 25(2):77-86, 1996.

52. Clark SR, Jones KD, Burckhardt CS, Bennett RM: Exercise for patients with fibromyalgia: risks versus benefits. *Curr Rheumatol Rep* 3(2):135-146, Apr 2001.

53. Jones KD, Clark SR, Bennett RM: Prescribing exercise for people with fibromyalgia. *AACN Clin Issues* 13(2):277-293, 2002.

54. Jones KD, Clark SR: Individualizing the exercise prescription for persons with fibromyalgia. *Rheum Dis Clin NA* 28:1-18, 2002.
Note: Videos of Jones and Clark's exercise programs for FMS patients, showing various levels of intensity can be ordered through *www.myalgia.com* with proceeds going to FMS research.

55. Sheperd C: Pacing and exercise in chronic fatigue syndrome. *Physiother* 87(8):395-396, Aug 2001.

56. Chaitow L: Soft-Tissue Manipulation: A Practitioner's Guide to the Diagnosis and Treatment of Soft Tissue Dysfunction and Reflex Activity. *Healing Arts Press*, Rochester, Vermont, 1988.

57. Travell JG, Simons DG: Myofascial Pain and Dysfunction: The Trigger Point Manual: Volume 1: The Upper Extremities. First Edition. *Williams & Wilkins*, Baltimore, 1983.

58. Travell JG, Simons DG: Myofascial Pain and Dysfunction. The Trigger Point Manual. Vol. 2: The Lower Extremities. First Edition. *Williams & Wilkins*, Baltimore, 1992.

59. Bennett RM: Emerging concepts in the neurobiology of chronic pain: evidence for abnormal sensory processing in fibromyalgia. *Mayo Clin Proceed* 74:385-398, 1999.

60. Weigent DA, Bradley LA, Blalock JE, Alarcon GS: Current concepts in the pathophysiology of abnormal pain perception in fibromyalgia. *Amer J Med Sci* 315(6):405-412, 1998.

61. Elert JE, Rantapaa Dahiqvist SB, Henriksson-Larsen K, Gerdle B: Increased EMG activity during short pauses in patients with primary fibromyalgia. *Scan J Rheum* 18:321-323, 1989.

62. Vaeroy H, Abrahamsen A, Forre O, Kass E: Treatment of fibromyalgia [fibrositis syndrome]: a parallel double blind trial with carisoprodol, paracetamol and caffeine [Somadril comp] versus placebo. *Clin Rheum* 8:245-250, 1989.

63. Bennett RM, [Treatment of Fibromyalgia with Ultracet]. Am J Med 114:537-545, 2003.

64. Russell IJ, Fletcher EM, Michalek JE, McBroom PC, Hester GG: Treatment of fibrositis/fibromyalgia syndrome with ibuprofen and alprazolam. A double-blind, placebo-controlled study. *Arthritis Rheum* 34:552-560, 1991.

65. Wassem R, McDonald M, Racine J: Fibromyalgia: patient perspectives on symptoms, symptom management, and provider utilization. *Clinic Nur Special* 16:24-28, 2002.

66. Goldenberg DL, Felson DT, Dinerman H: A randomized, controlled trial of amitriptyline and naproxen in the treatment of patients with fibromyalgia. *Arthritis Rheum* 29:1371-1377, 1986.

67. Simms RW, Felson DT, Goldenberg DL: Development of preliminary criteria for response to treatment in fibromyalgia syndrome. *J Rheumatol* 18:1558-1563, 1991.

68. Bayes MR: *Gateways to Clinical Trials*. June 2002. *Methods & Findings in Experimental & Clinical Pharmacol* 24:291-327, 2002.

69. Carette S: What have clinical trials taught us about treatment of fibromyalgia. Fibromyalgia, Chronic Fatigue Syndrome and Repetitive Injury: Current Concepts in Diagnosis, Management, Disability and Health Economics. Editors: Chalmers A, Littlejohn GO, Salit I, Wolfe F: *Haworth Medical Press*, Binghamton, NY 1995.

70. Carette S, Bell JJ, Reynolds WJ, Haraoui B, McCain GA, Bykerk VP: Comparison of amitriptyline, cyclobenzaprine, and placebo in the treatment of fibromyalgia: a randomized, double-blind clinical trial. *Arthritis Rheum* 37:32-40, 1994.

71. Carette S, Oakson G, Guimont C, Steriade M: Sleep electroencephalography and the clinical response to amitriptyline in patients with fibromyalgia. *Arthritis Rheum* 38:1211-1217, 1995.

72. Cathey MA, Wolfe F, Roberts FK, Bennett RM Caro X, Goldenberg DL: Demographic, work disability, service utilization and treatment characteristics of 620 fibromyalgia patients in rheumatologic practice. *Arthritis Rheum* 33;S10, 1990

73. Fors EAS: The effect of guided imagery and amitriptyline on daily fibromyalgia pain: a prospective,

randomized, controlled trial. *J Psychiat Research* 36: 179-187, 2002.

74. Forseth KK, Gran JT: Management of fibromyalgia: what are the best treatment choices? *Drugs* 62:577-592, 2002.

75. Gabriel SE, Bombardier C: Clinical trials in fibrositis: a critical review and future directions. *J Rheumatol* 19:177-179, 1989.

76. Godfrey RG: A guide to the understanding and use of tricyclic antidepressants in the overall management of fibromyalgia and other chronic pain syndromes. *Arch Intern Med* 1565:1047-1052, 1996.

77. Goldenberg D, Mayskly M, Mossey C, Ruthazer R, Schmid C: A randomized, double-blind crossover trial of fluoxetine and amitriptyline in the treatment of fibromyalgia. [Comment] *Arthritis Rheum* 39:1852-1859, 1996.

78. Jaeschke R, Adachi J, Guyatt G, Keller J, Wong B: Clinical usefulness of amitriptyline in fibromyalgia: the results of 23 N-of-1randomized controlled trials. *J Rheumatol* 18:447-451, 1991.

79. Godfrey RG: A guide to the understanding and use of tricyclic antidepressants in the overall management of fibromyalgia and other chronic pain syndromes. *Arch Intern Med* 156;1047-1052, 1996.

80. Romano TJ: Fibromyalgia in children; diagnosis and treatment. *W V Med J* 87:112-114, 1991.

81. Wassem R, McDonald M, Racine J: Fibromyalgia: patient perspectives on symptoms, symptom management, and provider utilization. *Clin Nur Special* 16: 24-28, 2002.

82. Bennett RM, Gatter RA, Campbell SM, Andrews RP, Clark SR, Scarola JA: A comparison of cyclobenzaprine and placebo in the management of fibrositis. A double-blind controlled study. *Arthritis Rheum* 31: 1535-1542, 1988.

83. Gatter RA: Pharmacotherapeutics in fibrositis. *Amer J Med* 81:63-66, 1986.

84. Goldenberg DL: Treatment of fibromyalgia syndrome. *Rheumat Dis Clin of NA* 15:61-71, 1989.

85. Quimby LG, Gratwick GM, Whitney CD, Block SR: A randomized trial of cyclobenzaprine for the treatment of fibromyalgia. *J Rhematol*–supplement 19: 140-143, 1989.

86. Reynolds, WJ, Moldofsky H, Saskin P, Lue FA: The effects of cyclobenzaprine on sleep physiology and symptoms in patients with fibromyalgia. *J Rheumatol* 18:452-454, 1991.

87. Arnold LM, Hess EV, Hudson JI, Welge JA, Berno SE, Keck PE, Jr: A randomized, placebo-controlled, double-blind, flexible-dose study of fluoxetine in the treatment of women with fibromyalgia [see comments]. *Amer J Med* 112:191-197, 2002.

88. Wolfe F, Cathey MA, Hawley DJ: A double-blind placebo controlled trial of fluoxetine in fibromyalgia. *Scand J Rheumatol* 23:255-259, 1994.

89. Goldstein GA: Betrayal by the Brain: The Neurological Basis of Chronic Fatigue Syndrome, Fibromyalgia Syndrome and Related Neural Network Disorders. *Haworth Medical Press*, Binghamton, NY, 1996

90. Selak I: Pregabalin [Pfizer]. *Cur Opin Investigational Drugs* 2:828-834, 2001.

91. Crofford L, Russell IJ, Mease P, Corbin A, Young J Jr, LaMoreaux L: Pregabalin improves pain associated with fibromyalgia syndrome in a multicenter, randomized, placebo-controlled monotherapy trial. *Arthritis Rheum* 46(9 Suppl, S613). 2002.

92. Farrar JT, Young JP Jr, Lamoreaux L, Werth JL, Poole RM: Clinical importance of changes in chronic pain intensity measured on an 11-point numerical pain rating scale. *Pain* 94:149-158, 2001.

93. Sorensen J, Bengsson A, Ahlner J, Henriksson KG, Ekselius L, Bengtsson M: Fibromyalgia–are there different mechanisms in the processing of pain? A double blind crossover comparison of analgesic drugs. *J Rheum* 24:1615-1621, 1997.

94. Kosek E, Ekholm J, Hansson P: Increased pressure pain sensibility in fibromyalgia patients is located deep to the skin but not restricted to muscle tissue. [Erratum appears in Pain 1996 Mar; 64(3):605.] *Pain* 63: 335-339, 1995.

95. Bennett MI, Tai YM: Intravenous lignocaine in the management of primary fibromyalgia syndrome. *Internat J Clin Pharmacol Research* 15:115-119, 1995.

96. Sorensen J, Bengtsson A, Backman E, Henriksson KG, Bengtsson M: Pain analysis in patients with fibromyalgia. Effects of intravenous morphine, lidocaine, and ketamine. *Scand J Rheumatol* 24:360-365, 1995.

97. Scudds RA, Janzen V, Delaney G, Heck C, McCain GA, Russell AL: The use of topical 4 percent lidocaine in sphenopalatine ganglion blocks for the treatment of chronic muscle pain syndromes: a randomized, controlled trial. *Pain* 62:69-77, 1995.

98. Caruso I, Sarzi Puttini P, Cazzola M, Azzolini V: Double-blind study of 5-hydroxytryptophan versus placebo in the treatment of primary fibromyalgia syndrome. *J Internat Med Research* 18:201-209, 1990.

99. Russell IJ, Vipraio GA, Acworth I: Abnormalities in the central nervous system [CNS] metabolism of tryptophan [TRY] to 3-hydroxy kynurenine [OHKY] in fibromyalgia syndrome. *Arthritis Rheum* 36(9):S222, 1993.

100. Freye E, Levy J: Acute abstinence syndrome following abrupt cessation of long-term use of tramadol [Ultram]: a case study. *Euro J Pain [EJP]* 4:307-3311, 2000.

101. Miller IJ, Kubes KL: Serotonergic agents in the treatment of fibromyalgia syndrome. [Review] [45 refs] *Annals of Pharmacother* 36:707-712, 2002.

102. Russell IJ, Kamin M, Bennett RM, Schnitzer TJ, Green JA, Katz WA: Efficacy of tramadol in treatment of pain in fibromyalgia. *J Clin Rheumatol* 6:250-257, 2000.

103. Graven-Nielsen T, Aspegren KS, Henriksson KG, Bengtsson M, Sorensen J, Johnson A: Ketamine reduces muscle pain, temporal summation, and referred pain in fibromyalgia patients. *Pain* 85:483-491, 2000.

104. Sorensen J, Bengtsson A, Backman E, Henriksson KG, Bengtsson M: Pain analysis in patients with fibromyalgia. Effects of intravenous morphine, lidocaine, and ketamine. *Scand J Rheumatol* 24:360-365, 1995.

105. Dalo NL, Larson AA: Effects of urethane and ketamine on substance P and excitatory amino acid-induced behavior in mice. *Euro J Pharmacol* 184:173-177, 1990.

106. Max MB, Byas-Smith MG, Gracely RH, Bennett GJ: Intravenous infusion of the NMDA antagonist, ketamine, in chronic posttraumatic pain with allodynia: a double-blind comparison to alfentanil and placebo. *Clin Neuropharmacol* 18:360-368, 1995.

107. Park KM, Max MB, Robinovitz E, Gracely RH, Bennett GJ: Effects of intravenous ketamine, alfentanil or placebo on pain, pinprick hyperalgesia, and allodynia produced by intradermal capsaicin in human subjects. *Pain* 63:163-172, 1995.

108. Dryson E: Venlafaxine and fibromyalgia. *NZ Med J* 113:87, 2000.

109. Dwight MM, Arnold LM, O'Brien H, Metzger R, Morris-Park E, Keck PE Jr: An open clinical trial of venlafaxine treatment of fibromyalgia. *Psychosomatics* 39:14-17, 1998.

110. Wallace DJ: Pyridostigmine for fibromyalgia: comment on the article by Paiva and a historical vignette. *Arthritis Rheum* 48:277-278, 2003.

111. Paiva ES, Deodhar A, Jones KD, Bennett RM: Impaired growth hormone secretion in fibromyalgia patients: evidence for augmented hypothalamic somatostatin tone. *Arthritis Rheum* 46:1344-1350, 2002.

112. May KP, West SG, Baker MR, Everett DW: Sleep apnea in male patients with the fibromyalgia syndrome. *Amer J Med* 94:505-508, 1993.

113. Pepin JL, Krieger J, Rodenstein D, Cornette A, Sforza E, Delguste P: Effective compliance during the first 3 months of continuous positive airway pressure. A European prospective study of 121 patients. *Amer J Respirat & Crit Care Med* 160:1124-1129, 1999.

114. Abbey NC, Cooper KR, Kwentus JA: Benefit of nasal CPAP in obstructive sleep apnea is due to positive pharyngeal pressure. *Sleep* 12;420-422, 1989.

115. Rapoport DM, Garay SM, Goldring RM: Nasal CPAP in obstructive sleep apnea: mechanisms of action. *Bull Euro de Physiopalologie Respiratoire* 19:616-620, 1983.

116. Biering-Sorensen F, Jacobsen E, Hjelms E, Fodstad H, Trojaborg W: [Diaphragm pacing by electric stimulation of the phrenic nerves.] [Danish] *Ugeskrift for Laeger* 152:1143-1145, 1990.

117. Wassem R, McDonald M, Racine J: Fibromyalgia: patient perspectives on symptoms, symptom management, and provider utilization. *Clin Nur Specialist* 16:24-28, 2002.

118. Moldofsky H, Lue FA, Mously C, Roth-Schechter B, Reynolds WJ: The effect of zolpidem in patients with fibromyalgia: a dose ranging, double blind, placebo controlled, modified crossover study. *J Rheumatol* 23:529-533, 1996.

119. Rothschild BM: Zolpidem efficacy in fibromyalgia. *J Rheumatol* 24:1012-1013, 1997.

120. Godfrey RG: A guide to the understanding and use of tricyclic antidepressants in the overall management of fibromyalgia and other chronic pain syndromes. *Arch Inter Med* 156:1047-1052, 1996.

121. Silva AB, Bertorini TE, Lemmi H: Polysomnography in idiopathic muscle pain syndrome [fibrositis]. *Arquivos de Neuro-Psiquiatria* 49:437-441, 1991.

122. Mitler MM, Browman CP, Menn SJ Gujavarty K, Timms RM: Nocturnal myoclonus: treatment efficacy of clonazepam and temazepam. *Sleep* 9:385-392, 1986.

123. Oshtory MA, Vijayan N: Clonazepam treatment of insomnia due to sleep myoclonus. *Arch Neurol* 37:119-120, 1980.

124. Bellometti S, Galzigna L: Function of the hypothalamic adrenal axis in patients with fibromyalgia syndrome undergoing mud-pack treatment. *Internat J Clin Pharmacol Resear* 19:27-33, 1999.

125. Saccomani L, Vigliarolo MA, Sbolgi P, Ruffa G, Doria LL: [Juvenile fibromyalgia syndrome: 2 clinical cases.] [Italian] *Pediatria Medica e Chirurgica* 15:99-101, 1993.

126. McLain D: An open-label, dose-finding trial of tizanidine [Zanaflex] for treatment of fibromyalgia. *J Musculoske Pain* 10(4):7-18, 2002.

127. Russell IJ, Michalek JE, Xiao Y, Haynes W, Vertiz R, Lawrence RA: Therapy with a central alpha-2-agonist [tizanidine] decreases cerebrospinal fluid substance P, and may reduce serum hyaluronic acid as it improves the clinical symptoms of the fibromyalgia syndrome. *Arthritis Rheum* 46:S614, 2002.

128. Lautenschlager J, Seglias J, Bruckle W, Muller W: Comparisons of spontaneous pain and tenderness in patients with primary fibromyalgia. *Clin Rheumatol* 10:168-173, 1991.

129. Staedt J, Wassmuth F, Ziemann U, Hajak G, Ruther E, Stoppe G: Pergolide: treatment of choice in restless legs syndrome [RLS] and nocturnal myoclonus syndrome [NMS]. A double-blind randomized crossover trial of pergolide versus L-Dopa. *J Neural Transmission* 104:461-468, 1997.

130. Rowe PC, Calkins H, DeBusk K, McKenzie R, Anand R, Sharma G, Cuccherini BA, Soto N, Hohman P, Snader S, Lucas KE, Wolff M, Straus SE: Fludocortisone acetate to treat neurally mediated hypotension in chronic fatigue syndrome: a randomized controlled trial. *JAMA* 285:52-59, 2001.

131. Baschetti R: Overlap of chronic fatigue syndrome with primary adrenocortical insufficiency. *Horm Metabol Research* 31:439, 1999.

132. Peterson PK, Pheley A, Schroeppel J, Schenck C, Marshall P, Kind A, Haugland JM, Lambrecht LJ, Swan S, Goldsmith S: A preliminary placebo-controlled crossover trial of fludrocortisone for chronic fatigue syndrome. *Arch Intern Med* 158:908-914, 1998.

133. Bou-Holaigah I, Rowe PC, Kan J, Calkins H: The relationship between neurally mediated hypotension

and the chronic fatigue syndrome. *JAMA* 274:961-967, 1995.

134. Kaufmann H, Saadia D, Voustianiouk A: Midodrine in neurally mediated syncope: a double-blind, randomized, crossover study. *Ann Neurol* 52:342-345, 2002.

135. Clissold SP, Heel RC: Transdermal hyoscine [Scopolamine]. A preliminary review of its pharmacodynamic properties and therapeutic efficacy. *Drugs* 29: 189-207, 1985.

136. Poynard T, Regimbeau C, Benhamou Y: Meta-analysis of smooth muscle relaxants in the treatment of irritable bowel syndrome. *Aliment Pharmacol Therapeut* 15:355-361, 2001.

137. Lu CL, Chen CY, Chang FY, Chang SS, Kang LJ, Lu RH, Lee SD: Effect of a calcium channel blocker and antispasmodic in diarrhea-predominant irritable bowel syndrome. *J Gastroenterol Hepatol* 15:925-930, 2000.

138. Bouchoucha M, Faye A, Devroede G, Arsac M: Effects of oral pinaverium bromide on colonic response to food in irritable bowel syndrome patients. *Biomed Parmacother* 54:381-387, 2000.

139. Awad RA, Cordova VH, Dibildox M, Santiago R, Camacho S: Reduction of post-prandial motility by pinaverium bromide a calcium channel blocker acting selectively on the gastrointestinal tract in patients with irritable bowel syndrome. *Acta Gastroenterol Latinoamericana* 27:247-251, 1997.

140. Awad R, Dibildox M, Ortiz F: Irritable bowel syndrome treatment using pinaverium bromide as a calcium channel blocker. A randomized double-blind placebo-controlled trial. *Acta Gastroenterol Latinoamericana* 25:137-144, 1995.

141. Poynard T, Naveau S, Mory B, Chaput JC: Meta-analysis of smooth muscle relaxants in the treatment of irritable bowel syndrome. *Aliment Pharmacol Therapeut* 8:499-510, 1994.

142. Bouchoucha M, Salles JP, Fallet M, Frileux P, Cugnenc PH, Barbier JP: Effect of pinaverium bromide on jejunal motility and colonic transit time in healthy humans. *Biomed Pharmacother* 46:161-165, 1992.

143. Christen MO: Action of pinaverium bromide, a calcium-antagonist, on gastrointestinal motility disorder. *General Pharmacol* 21:821-825, 1990.

144. Passaretti S, Sorghi M, Colombo E, Mazzotti G, Tittobello A, Guslandi M: Motor effects of locally administered pinaverium bromide in the sigmoid tract of patients with irritable bowel syndrome. *Internat J Clin Pharmacol, Ther Toxicol* 27:47-50, 1989.

145. Fioramonti J, Prexinos J, Staumont G, Bueno L: Inhibition of the colonic motor response to eating by pinaverium bromide in irritable bowel syndrome patients. *Fundament Clin Pharmacol* 2:19-27, 1988.

146. Poynard T, Regimbeau C, Benhamou Y: Meta-analysis of smooth muscle relaxants in treatment of irritable bowel syndrome. *Aliment Pharmacol Therapeut* 15:355-361, 2001.

147. Ritchie JA, Truelove SC: Comparison of various treatments for irritable bowel syndrome. *Brit Med J* 281:1317-1319, 1980.

148. Ritchie JA, Truelove SC: Treatment of irritable bowel syndrome with lorazepam, hyoscine butylbromide, and ispaghula husk. *Brit Med J* 1:376-378, 1979.

149. Barbalias GA, Liatsikos EN, Athanoasopoulos A, Nidiforidis G: Interstitial cystitis: bladder training with intravesical oxybutynin. *J Urol* 163:1818-1822, 2000.

150. Haeusler G, Leitich H, van Trotsenburg M, Kaider A, Tempfer CB: Drug therapy of urinary urge incontinence: a systematic review. *Obstet Gynecol* 100: 1003-1016, 2002.

151. Cardozo LD, Stanton SL: An objective comparison of the effects of parenterally administered drugs in patients suffering from detrusor instability. *J Urol* 122: 58-59, 1979.

152. Wang PS, Levin R, Zhao SZ, Avorn J: Urinary antispasmodic use of the risks of ventricular arrhythmia and sudden death in older patients. *J Amer Geriat Soc* 50:117-124, 2002.

153. Sevenoaks M, Gorard DA: Jaundice associated with flavoxate. *J Amer Geriat Soc* 92:589, 1999.

154. Kimura Y, Sasaki Y, Hamada K, Fukui H, Ukai Y, Yoshikuni Y, Kimura K, Sugaya K, Nishizawa O: Mechanisms of the suppression of the bladder activity by flavoxate. *Internat J Urol* 3:218-227, 1996.

155. Caine M, Gin S, Pietra C, Ruffmann R: Antispasmodic effects of flavoxate, MFCA, and REC 15/2053 on smooth muscle of human prostate and urinary bladder. *Urol* 37:390-394, 1991.

156. Chapple CR, Parkhouse H, Gardener C, Milroy EJ: Double-blind, placebo-controlled, cross-over study of flavoxate in the treatment of idiopathic detrusor instability. *Brit J Urol* 66:491-494, 1990.

157. Russell IJ, Fletcher EM, Michalek JE, McBroom PC, Hester GG: Treatment of primary fibrositis/fibromyalgia syndrome with ibuprofen and alprazolam. A double-blind, placebo-controlled study. *Arthritis Rheum* 34:552-560, 1991.

158. Paira SO: Fibromyalgia associated with female urethral syndrome. *Clin Rheumatol* 13:88-89, 1994.

159. Bymaster FP, Zhang W, Carter PA, Shaw J, Chernet E, Phebus L, Wong DT, Perry KW: Fluoxetine, but not other selective serotonin uptake inhibitors, increases norepinephrine and dopamine extracellular levels in prefrontal cortex. *Psychopharmacol* 160:353-361, 2002.

160. Maes M, Libbrecht I, Delmeire L, Lin A, De Clerck L, Scharpe S, Janca A: Changes in platelet alpha-2-adrenoceptors in fibromyalgia: effects of treatment with antidepressants. *Neuropsychobiol* 40:129-133, 1999.

161. Maes M, Libbrecht I, Van Hunsel F, Lin AH, Bonaccorso S, Goossens F: Lower serum activity of prolyl endopeptidase in fibromyalgia is related to severity of depressive symptoms and pressure hyperalgesia. *Pycholog Med* 28:957-965, 1998.

162. Anderberg UM, Marteinsdottir I, von Knorring L: Citalopram in patients with fibromyalgia–a randomized, double-blind, placebo-controlled study. *Euro J Pain [EJP]* 4:27-35, 2000.

163. Keller MB, Ryan ND, Strober M, Klein RG, Kutcher SP Birmaher B: Efficacy of paroxetine in the treatment of adolescent major depression: a randomized, controlled trial. [Comment] *J Amer Acad Child Adoles Psychia* 40:762-772, 2001.

164. Waldinger MD, van De Pa, Pattij T, van Oorschot R, Coolen LM, Veening JG, Olivier B: The selective serotonin re-uptake inhibitors fluvoxamine and paroxetine differ in sexual inhibitory effects after chronic treatment. *Psychopharmacol* 160:283-289, 2002.

165. Itil TM, Shrivastava RK, Mukherjee S, Coleman BS, Michael ST: A double-blind placebo-controlled study of fluvoxamine and imipramine in out-patients with primary depression. *Br J Clin Pharm* 15 Suppl 3:433-438S, 1983.

166. Hacket GS, Hermwall GA, Montgomery GA: Ligament and Tendon Relaxation Treatment by Prolotherapy. *Institute of Basic Life Principles* 1993.

167. Reeves KD: Treatment of consecutive severe fibromyalgia patients with prolotherapy. *J Orthopaedic Med* 16:84-89, 1994.

168. Gunn CC: The Gunn Approach to the Treatment of Chronic Pain. *Churchill Livingstone*, New York, Edinburgh, London, Madrid, Melbourne, San Francisco, Tokyo 1996.

169. Silverstone LM: The use of a new, non-invasive, neuromodulation device in the treatment of acute and chronic pain. [Abstract] [presented at the First Scientific Meeting of the American Neuromodulation Society], Orlando FL, Mar 6-8, 1996

170. Torlage RJ, What's new in 2001? Sota Instruments. Aug 31 2001. *http://www.sotainstruments.com*

171. Romano T: Exacerbation of soft tissue rheumatism by vitamin A excess. *WV Med J* (91):147, 1995.

172. Abraham GE, Flechas JD: Management of fibromyalgia: Rationale for the use of magnesium and malic acid. *J Nutrit Med* 3:49-59, 1992.

173. Russell IH, Michalek JE, MacKillip F, Lopez YM, Abraham GE: Treatment of fibromyalgia syndrome with malic acid and magnesium: A randomized, double-blind, placebo-controlled, cross-over study. *J Rheumatol* 22:953-958, 1995.

174. Clauw D, Ward K, Katz P, Rajan S: Muscle intracellular magnesium levels correlate with pain tolerance in fibromyalgia [FM]. *Arthritis Rheum* 37(Suppl): S29, 1994.

175. Neeck G, Riedel W: Thyroid function in patients with fibromyalgia syndrome. *J Rheumatol* 19:1120-1122, 1992.

176. Ng SY: Hair calcium and magnesium levels in patients with fibromyalgia: a case center study. *J Manipulat Physio Ther* 22(9):586-593, 1999.

177. Crofford LJ, Pillemer SR, Kalogeras KT, Cash JM, Michelson D, Kling MA: Hypothalamic-pituitary-adrenal axis perturbations in patients with fibromyalgia. *Arthritis Rheum* 37:1583-1592, 1994.

178. Kang Y-K, Russell IJ, Vipraio GA, Acworth IN: Low urinary 5-hydroxyindole acetic acid in fibromyalgia syndrome: evidence in support of a serotonin-deficiency pathogenesis. *Myalgia* 1:14-21, 1998.

179. Russell IJ: Advances in fibromyalgia: possible role for central neurochemicals. *Am J Med Sci* 315(6): 377-384, 1998.

180. Rau C-L, Russell IJ: Is Fibromyalgia a distinct clinical syndrome? *Cur Rev Pain* 4(4):287-294, 2000.

181. Russell IJ: Is fibromyalgia a distinct clinical entity? The clinical investigator's evidence. *Best Pract & Res Clin Rheum* 13:445-454, 1999.

182. Russell IJ: San Antonio, Texas, 1990, Unpublished.

183. Yunus M, Khan MA, Rawlings KK, Green JR, Olson JM, Shuhrat S: Genetic linkage analysis of multicase families with fibromyalgia syndrome. *J Rheumatol* 26:408-412, 1999.

184. Buskila D, Neumann L, Hazanov I, Carmi R: Familial aggregation in the fibromyalgia syndrome. *Semin Arthritis Rheum* 26:605-611, 1996.

185. Roizenblatt S, Feldman DF, Goldenberg J, Tufik S: Juvenile fibromyalgia-infant-mother association. *J Musculoske Pain* 3(Suppl #3):118, 1995.

186. Green JR, Shah S: Power comparison of various sibship tests of association. *Ann Hum Genet* 57:151-158, 1993.

187. Deloukas P, Schuler GD, Gyapay G, Beasley EM, Soderlund C, Rodriguez-Tome P: A physical map of 30,000 human genes. *Science* 282:744-746, 1998.

188. Lander ES, Linton LM, Birren B, Nusbaum C, Zody MC, Baldwin J, International Human Genome Sequencing Consortium: Initial sequencing and analysis of the human genome. *Nature* 409:860-921, 2001.

189. McPherson JD, Marra M, Hillier L, Waterston RH, Chinwalla A, Wallis J, Internat Human Genome Mapping Consortium: A physical map of the human genome. *Nature* 409:934-941.

190. Greenfield S, Fitzcharles MA, Esdaile JM: Reactive fibromyalgia syndrome. *Arthritis Rheum* 35: 678-681, 1992.

191. Bennett RM: Disabling fibromyalgia: appearance versus reality. *J Rheumatol* 20:1821-1824, 1993.

192. Moldofsky H, Wong MT, Lue FA: Litigation, sleep, symptoms and disabilities in post accident pain [fibromyalgia]. *J Rheumatol* 20:1935-1940, 1993.

193. Pellegrino MJ: Post-traumatic Fibromyalgia: a Medical Perspective. Columbus, Ohio: *Anadem Publishing*, 1996.

194. Wolfe F: Post-traumatic fibromyalgia: a case report narrated by the patient. *Arth Care Res* 7:161-165, 1994.

195. Buskila D, Neumann L, Vaisberg G, Alkalay D, Wolfe F: Increased rate of fibromyalgia following cervical spine injury. A controlled study of 161 cases of traumatic injury. *Arthritis Rheum* 40:446, 1997.

196. Weinberger LM: Traumatic fibromyositis: a critical review of an enigmatic concept. *West J Med* 127:99, 1977.

197. Romano TJ: Clinical experience with post-traumatic fibromyalgia syndrome. *WV Med J* 86:198-202, 1990.

198. Saskin P, Moldofsky H, Lue FA: Sleep and post-traumatic rheumatic pain modulation disorder [fibrositis syndrome]. *Psychosom Med* 48:319-323, 1986.

199. Waylonis GW, Perkins RH: Post-traumatic fibromyalgia. A long-term follow-up. *Amer J Phys Med Rehab* 73(6):403-412, 1994.

200. Wolfe F: The clinical syndrome of fibrositis. *Amer J Med* 8(Suppl 3A):7-14, 1986.

201. Johnson G: Hyperextension soft tissue injuries of cervical spine–a review. *J Acc Emerg Med* 13(1): 3-8, 1996.

202. Claussen CF, Claussen E: Neurootological contribution to the diagnostic follow-up after whiplash injuries. *Acta Otolaryngol* [Stockh] (Suppl) 520:53-56, 1995.

203. Pettersson K, Karrholm J, Toolanen G, Hildingsson C: Decreased width of the spinal canal in patients with chronic symptoms after whiplash injury. *Spine* 20(15): 1664-1667, 1995.

204. Hamer AJ, Gargan MF, Bannister GC, Nelson RJ: Whiplash injury and surgically treated cervical disc disease. *Injury* 24(8):549-550, 1993.

205. Heffez DS, Malone DG, Banner SR, Shepard A, Ross RE, Robertson JW: Can spinal cord compression cause fibromyalgia syndrome? *National Fibromyalgia Research Foundation Conference* in Portland, Oregon–Sept 26-27, 1999.

206. Alarcon GS, Bradley LA, Hadley MN, Sotolongo A, Alberts KR, Martin MY: Does Chiari Malformation contribute to fibromyalgia [FM] symptoms? *1997 American College of Rheumatology Meeting*, Abstract No. 953.

207. Yunus MB, Bennett RM, Romano TJ, Russell IJ : Fibromyalgia Consensus Report: Additional Comments. *J Clin Rheum* 3(6): 3324-3327, 1997.

208. Hudson JI, Hudson MS, Pliner LF, Goldenberg DL, Pope HG, Jr: Fibromyalgia and major affective disorder: a controlled phenomenology and family history study. *Amer J Psychia* 142:441-446, 1985.

209. Ahles TA, Khan SA, Yunus MB, Spiegel DA, Masi AT: Psychiatric status of patients with primary fibromyalgia, patients with rheumatoid arthritis, and subjects without pain: a blind comparison of DSM-III diagnoses. *Amer J Psychia* 148:1721-1726, 1991.

210. Kirmayer LJ, Robbins JM, Kapusta MA: Somatization and depression in fibromyalgia syndrome. *Am J Psychia* 145:950-954, 1988.

211. Galloway J: Maintaining serenity in chronic illness. *NY State J Med* 90:366-367, 1990.

212. Yunus MB: Psychological aspects of fibromyalgia syndrome: a component of the dysfunctional spectrum syndrome. *Baillieres Clin Cheumatol* 9:811-837, 1994.

213. Goldenberg DL: Psychological symptoms and psychiatric diagnosis in patients with fibromyalgia. *J Rheumatol Suppl* 19:127-130, 1989.

214. Ward MM: Are patient self-report measures of arthritis activity confounded by mood? A longitudinal study of patients with rheumatoid arthritis. *J Rheumatol* 21:1046-1050, 1994.

215. Maes M, Lin A, Bonaccorso S, Van Hunsel F, Van Gastel A, Delmeire L: Increased 24-hour urinary cortisol excretion in patients with post-traumatic stress disorder and patients with major depression, but not in patients with fibromyalgia. *Acta Psychiatrica Scand* 98: 328-335, 1998.

216. Hudson JI, Pliner LF, Hudson MS, Goldenberg DL, Melby JC: The dexamethasone suppression test in fibrositis. *Biolog Psychia* 19:1489-1493, 1984.

217. Neeck G, Riedel W: Hormonal perturbations in fibromyalgia syndrome. *Ann NY Acad Sci* 876:325-338, 1999.

218. Griep EN, Boersma JW, de Kloet ER: Altered reactivity of the hypothalamic-pituitary-adrenal axis in the primary fibromyalgia syndrome. *J Rheumatol* 20: 469-474, 1993.

219. Russell IJ, Orr MD, Littman B, Vipraio GA, Alboukrek D, Michalek JE: Elevated cerebrospinal levels of substance P in patients with the fibromyalgia syndrome. *Arthritis Rheum* 37:1593-1601, 1994.

220. Martensson B, Nyberg S, Toresson G, Brodin E, Bertilsson L: Fluoxetine treatment of depression. Clinical effects, drug concentrations and monoamine metabolites and N-terminally extended substance P in cerebrospinal fluid. *Acta Psychia Scand* 79:586-596, 1989.

221. Yunus MB: Fibromyalgia syndrome: clinical features and spectrum. *J Musculoskel Pain* 2(3):5-21, 1994.

222. Veale D, Kavanagh G, Fielding JF, Fitzgerald O: Primary fibromyalgia and the irritable bowel syndrome: different expressions of a common pathogenetic process. *Br J Rheumol* 30:220-222, 1991.

223. Finestone HM, Stenn P, Davies F, Stalker C, Fry R, Koumanis J: Chronic pain and health care utilization in women with a history of childhood sexual abuse. *Child Abuse Neglect* 24:547-556, 2000.

224. Goldberg RT, Pachas WN, Keith D: Relationship between traumatic events in childhood and chronic pain. *Disabil Rehab* 21:23-30, 1999.

225. Russell IJ, Russell SJ, Cuevas RE, Michalek JE: Early life traumas and confiding in fibromyalgia syndrome. *Scand J Rheumatol* 94:S14, 1992.

226. Hudson JI, Pope HG, Jr: Does childhood sexual abuse cause fibromyalgia? *Arthritis Rheum* 38:161-163, 1995.

227. Rapheal KG, Marbach JJ: Widespread pain and the effectiveness of oral splints in myofascial face pain. *J Amer Dent Assoc* 132:305-316, 2001.

228. Moldofsky H: Fibromyalgia, sleep disorder and chronic fatigue syndrome. *Ciba Foundation Symposium* 173:262-279, 1993.

229. Lue F, MacLean A, Moldofsky H: Sleep physiology and psychological aspects of the fibrositis [fibromyalgia] syndrome. *Can J Psych* 45(2):179-184, 1991.

230. Harding SM: Sleep in fibromyalgia patients: subjective and objective findings. *Amer J Med Sci* 315: 367-376, 1998.

231. Martinez-Lavin M, Hermosillo AG, Rosas M, Soto ME: Circadian studies of autonomic nervous balance in patients with fibromyalgia: a heart rate variability analysis. *Arthritis Rheum* 41(11):1966-1971, 1998.

232. Zidar J, Backman E, Bengtsson A, Henrickson KG: Quantitative EMG and muscle tension in painful muscles in fibromyalgia. *Pain* 40:249-254, 1990.

233. Liller TK, Mutter JB, Catlett JL: Fibromyalgia: a multi-dimensional profile. *Fibromyalgia Association of Greater Washington, Inc.* Fairfax, VA, pp. 71-76, 1995.

234. Plesh O, Wolfe F, Lane N: The relationship between fibromyalgia and temporomandibular disorders: prevalence and symptom severity. *J Rheumatol* 23: 1948-1952, 1996.

235. Evaskus DS, Laskin DM: A biochemical measure of stress in patients with myofascial pain dysfunction syndrome. *J Dent Res* 1972;51:1464-1466, 1972.

236. Fricton JR, Kroening R, Haley D: Myofascial pain syndrome of the head and neck: a review of clinical characteristics of 164 patients. *Oral Surg Oral Med Oral Pathol* 60:615-623, 1985.

237. Ware JC: Nocturnal myoclonus: possible mediation by the sympathetic nervous system. [Abstract] *Sleep Resear* 14:24, 1985.

238. MacFarlane JG, Shahal B, Mously C, Moldofsky H: Periodic K-alpha sleep EEG activity and periodic limb movements during sleep: comparisons of clinical features and sleep parameters. *Sleep* 19:200-204, 1996.

239. Glass JM, Park DC: Cognitive dysfunction in fibromyalgia. *Cur Rheumatol Reports* 3(2):123-127, 2001.

240. Turk DC, Okifuji A: Evaluating the role of physical, operant, cognitive, and affective factors in the pain behaviors of chronic pain patients. *Behav Modific* 21: 259-280, 1997.

241. Grace GM, Nielson WR, Hopkins M, Berg MA: Concentrations and memory deficits in patients with fibromyalgia syndrome. *J Clin Exper Neuropsychol* 21: 477-487, 1999.

242. Cote KA, Moldofsky H: Sleep, daytime symptoms, and cognitive performance in patients with fibromyalgia. *J Rheumatol* 24:2014-2023, 1997.

243. Sarnoch H, Adler F, Scholz OB: Relevance of muscular sensitivity, muscular activity, and cognitive variables for pain reduction associated with EMG biofeedback in fibromyalgia. *Percept Motor Skills* 84: 1043-1050, 1997.

244. Sherkey J: The neurological basis of chronic fatigue syndrome & fibromyalgia. [Synopsis of Betrayal by the Brain: the Neurological Basis of Chronic Fatigue Syndrome, Fibromyalgia and Related Neural Network Disorder by J. Goldstein.] ME & FMS Conference in Sudbury, ON. Sept 1997.

245. Donaldson CCS, Sella GE, Mueller HH: Fibromyalgia: a retrospective study of 252 consecutive referrals. *Can J Clin Med* 5(6):116-127, June 1998.

246. Moldofsky H: Non-restorative sleep and symptoms after a febrile illness in patients with fibrositis and chronic fatigue syndrome. *J Rheumatol* (Suppl) 19: 150S-153S, 1989.

247. Anch AM, Lue FA, MacLean AW, Moldofsky H: Sleep physiology and psychological aspects of the fibrositis [fibromyalgia] syndrome. *C J Psychol* 45: 179-184, 1991.

248. Michiels V, Chuydts R, Fischler B: Attention and verbal learning in patients with chronic fatigue syndrome. *J Int Neuropsychol Soc* 4(5)456-466, 1998.

249. McDermid AJ, Rollman GB, McCain GA: Generalized hypervigilance in Fibromyalgia: evidence of perceptual amplification. *Pain* 66:133-144, 1996.

250. Lautenbacher S, Rollman GB, MaCain GA: Multi-method assessment of experimental and clinical pain in patients with fibromyalgia. *Pain* 59:45-53, 1994.

251. Goldstein JA: Chronic Fatigue Syndromes: The Limbic Hypothesis. *Haworth Medical Press*, Binghamton, New York, 1993, p. 42

252. Slotkoff AT, Radulovic DA, Clauw DJ: The relationship between fibromyalgia and multiple chemical sensitivity syndrome. *Scand J Rheumatol* 26(5):364-367, 1997.

253. Goldenberg DL: Fibromyalgia and its relation to chronic fatigue syndrome, viral illness and immune abnormalities. *J Rheumatol* 9:91-93, 1989.

254. Goldenberg DL: Fibromyalgia, chronic fatigue, and myofascial pain syndromes. *Curr Opin Rheum* 4: 247-257, 1992.

255. Reilly PA, Littlejohn GO: Fibromyalgia and chronic fatigue syndrome. *Curr Opin Rheum* 2:282-290, 1990.

256. Clauw DJ: The pathogenesis of chronic pain and fatigue syndromes, with special reference to fibromyalgia. *Med Hypoth* 44:369-378, 1995.

257. Buskila D: Fibromyalgia, chronic fatigue syndrome, and myofascial pain syndrome. *Curr Opin Rheum* 13:117-127, 2001.

258. Steinberg AD: On morning stiffness. *J Rheumatol* 5:3-6, 1978.

259. Hazes JMW, Hayton R, Silman AJ: A reevaluation of the symptom of morning stiffness. *J Rheumatol* 20:1138-1142, 1993.

260. Buchanan WW: Assessment of joint tenderness, grip strength, digital joint circumference and morning stiffness in rheumatoid arthritis. *J Rheumatol* 9:763-766, 1982.

261. Arnett FC: The American Rheumatism Association 1987 revised criteria for the classification of rheumatoid arthritis. *Arthritis Rheum* 31:315, 1994.

262. Pinal RS, Massi AT, Larse RA: Preliminary criteria for clinical remission of rheumatoid arthritis. *Arthritis Rheum* 24:1308-1315, 1981.

263. Engstrom-Laurent A, Hällgren R: Circulating hyaluronic acid levels vary with physical activity in

healthy subjects and in rheumatoid arthritis patients. Relationship to synovitis mass and morning stiffness. *Arthritis Rheum* 30:1333-1338, 1987.

264. Thompson S, Kelly CA, Griffiths ID, Turner GA: Abnormally-fucosylated serum haptoglobins in patients with inflammatory joint disease. *Clinica Chimica Acta* 184:251-258, 1989.

265. Azzini M, Girelli D, Olivieri O, Guarini P, Stganzial AM, Frigo A: Fatty acids and antioxidant micronutrients in psoriatic arthritis. *J Rheumatol* 22: 103-108, 1995.

266. Yaron M, Buskila D, Shire D, Neumann L, Elkind-Hirsch K, Paredes W: Elevated levels of hyaluronic acid in the sera of women with fibromyalgia. *J Rheumatol* 24:2221-2224,1997.

267. Balblanc JC, Hartmann D, Noyer D, Mathieu P, Conrozier T, Tron AM : [Serum hyaluronic acid in osteoarthritis.] [French]. *Revue du Rhumatisme* Edition Francaise 194-202, 1993.

268. Yoshinoya S, Mizoguchi Y, Hashimoto Y, Yamada A, Uchida S, Taniguchi A : [Serum concentration of hyaluronic acid in healthy populations and patients with rheumatoid arthritis–relationship to clinical disease activity of RA.] [Japanese] *Ryumachi* 31:381-390, 1991.

269. Lindman R, Hagberg M, Bengtsson A, Henriksson KG, Thornell L-E: Capillary structure and mitochonrial volume density in the trapezius muscle of chronic trapezius myalgia, fibromyalgia and healthy subjects. *J Musculoske Pain* 3(3):5-22, 1995

270. Bengtsson A, Henriksson KG, Larsson J: Reduced high energy phosphate levels in the painful muscles of patients with primary fibromyalgia. *Arthritis Rheum* 29:817-821, 1986.

271. Lund N, Bengtsson A, Thorberg P: Muscle tissue oxygen pressure in primary fibromyalgia. *Scand J Rheumatol* 15:165-173, 1986.

272. Simms RW: Is there muscle pathology in fibromyalgia syndrome? *Rheum Dis Clin NA* 22:245-266, 1996.

273. Vestergaard-Poulsen P, Thomsen C, Norregaard J, Bulow P, Sinkjaer T, Henriksen O: ^{31}P NMR spectroscopy and electromyography during exercise and recovery in patients with fibromyalgia. *J Rheumatol* 22: 1544-1551, 1995.

274. Yunus MB, Kalyan-Raman UP, Masi AT, Aldag JC: Electron microscopic studies of muscle biopsy in primary fibromyalgia syndrome: A controlled and blinded study. *J Rheumatol* 16:97-101, 1989.

275. Frey LD, Locher JT, Hrycaj P, Stratz T, Kovac C, Mennet P, Muller W: [Determination of regional rate of glucose metabolism in lumbar muscles in patients with generalized tendomyopathy using dynamic 18F-FDG PET.] [German] *Z Rheumatol* 51:238-242, 1992.

276. Simons DG: Myofascial trigger points: a need for understanding. *Arch Phys Med Rehabil* 62:97-99, 1981.

277. Granges G, Littlejohn G: Prevalence of myofascial pain syndrome in fibromyalgia syndrome and regional pain syndrome: a comparative study. *J Musculoske Pain* 1(2):19-36, 1993.

278. Hong C-Z, Hsueh T-C, Simons DG: Difference in pain relief after trigger point injections in myofascial pain patients with and without fibromyalgia. *J Musculoske Pain* 3(suppl 1):60, 1995.

279. Elert JE, Rantapaa-Dahlqvist SB, Henriksson-Larsen K, Lorentzon R, Gerdle BU: Muscle performance, electromyography and fibre type composition in fibromyalgia and work-related myalgia. *Scand J Rheumatol* 21:28-34, 1992.

280. Elert J, Gerdle B: The relationship between contraction and relaxation during fatiguing isokinetic shoulder flexions. An electromyographic study. *Euro J Appl Physiol & Occup Physiol* 59:303-309, 1989.

281. Mengshoel AM, Komnaes HB, Forre O: The effects of 20 weeks of physical fitness training in female patients with fibromyalgia. *Clin Exp Rheumatol* 10: 345-349, 1992.

282. Jacobsen S, Holm B: Muscle strength and endurance compared to aerobic capacity in primary fibromyalgia syndrome. *Clin Exp Rheumatol* 10:419-427, 1992.

283. Jacobsen S, Hoydalsmo OJ: Experiment or research on muscle physiology during work and exercise. Progress in fibromyalgia and myofascial pain. *Pain Resear & Clin Manag* 6, 1993. Amsterdam: *Elsevier Science Publishers.*

284. Bennett RM, Clark SR, Campbell SM, Burckhardt CS: Low levels of somatomedin C in patients with the fibromyalgia syndrome: a possible link between sleep and muscle pain. *Arthritis Rheum* 35:1113-1116, 1992.

285. Riek S, Chapman AE, Milner T: A simulation of muscle force and internal kinematics of extensor carpi radialis brevis during backhand tennis stroke: implication for injury. *Clin Biomech* 14:477-483, 1999.

286. Saxon L, Finch C, Bass S: Sports participation, sports injuries and osteoarthritis: implications for prevention. *Sports Med* 28:123-135, 1999.

287. Bauer JA, Murray RD: Electromyographic patterns of individuals suffering from lateral tennis elbow. *J Electromyogr Kinesiol* 9:245-252, 1999.

288. Sun JS, Hou SM, Hang YS, Liu TK, Lu KS: Ultrastructural studies on myofibrillogenesis and neogenesis of skeletal muscles after prolonged traction in rabbits. *Histol Histopath* 11:285-292, 1996.

289. Hutchins MO, Skjonsby HS: Microtrauma to rat superficial masseter muscles following lengthening contractions. *J Dent Resear* 69:1580-1585, 1990.

290. Bennett RM: Beyond fibromyalgia: ideas on etiology and treatment. *J Rheumatol* 19(Suppl):185-191, 1989.

291. Bonica JJ: Definitions and Taxonomy of Pain. In: The Management of Pain, Vol. 1, 2nd edition. Edited by Bonica JJ, Loeser JD, Chapmanand CR, Fordyce WE. *Lea & Febiger*, Philadelphia, 1990, pp. 18-27.

292. Russell IJ: Neurochemical pathogenesis of fibromyalgia syndrome. *J Musculoske Pain* 1(1&2):61-92, 1996.

293. McCain GA: The clinical features of the fibromyalgia syndrome. In: Pain Research and Clinical Management. *Anonymous Elsevier Science Publishers*, Amsterdam, 1993.

294. Terman GW, Bonica JJ: Spinal Mechanisms and Their Modulation. In: Bonica's Management of Pain. Third edition. Edited by Loeser JD, Butler SH, Chapmanand CR, Turk DC. *Lippincott Williams & Wilkins*, Philadelphia, PA, 2001, pp. 73-152.

295. Malmberg AB, Yaksh TL: Hyperalgesia mediated by spinal glutamate or substance P receptor blocked by spinal cyclooxygenase inhibition. *Science* 257: 1276-1279, 1992.

296. Hoheisel U, Mense S, Ratkai M: Effects of spinal cord superfusion with substance P on the excitability of rat dorsal horn neurons processing input from deep tissues. *J Musculoske Pain* 3(3):23-43, 1995.

297. Fischer HP, Hierl T, Werle E, Freitag C, Eich W: Substance P in saliva and serum of patients with fibromyalgia syndrome and rheumatoid arthritis. Unpublished.

298. Schwarz MJ, Spath M, Muller-Bardorff H, Pongratz DE, Bondy B, Ackenheil M: Relationship of substance P, 5-hydroxyindole acetic acid, and tryptophan in serum of fibromyalgia patients. *Neurosci Lett* 259:196-198, 1999.

299. Vaeroy H, Helle R, Forre O, Kass E, Terenius L: Elevated CSF levels of substance P and high incidence of Raynaud's phenomenon in patients with fibromyalgia: new features for diagnosis. *Pain* 32:21-26, 1988.

300. Welin M, Bragee B, Nyberg F, Kristiansson M: Elevated substance P levels are contrasted by a decrease in met-enkephalin-arg-phe levels in CSF from fibromyalgia patients. *J Musculoske Pain* 3(Suppl 1):4, 1995.

301. Bradley LA, Alberts KR, Alarcon GS, Alexander MT, Mountz JM, Weigent DA: Abnormal brain regional cerebral blood flow [rCBF] and cerebrospinal fluid [CSF] levels of substance P [SP] in patients and non-patients with fibromyalgia [FM]. *Arthritis Rheum* 39(Suppl):S212, 1996.

302. Russell IJ, Fletcher EM, Vipraio GA, Lopez Y, Orr MA: Cerebrospinal fluid [CSF] substance P [SP] in fibromyalgia: changes in CSF SP over time parallel changes in clinical activity. *J Musculoske Pain* 6(Suppl 2):77, 1998.

303. Alberts KR, Bradley LA, Mountz JM, Blalock JE, Jiu JG, Weigent DA: Regional cerebral blood flow [rCBF] in the caudate nucleus and thalamus of fibromyalgia [RM] patients is associated with the cerebrospinal fluid [CSF] levels of substance P [SP]. [Abstract] 8th World Congress on Pain, Aug 17-22. *IASP Press*, Seattle, WA 445, 1996.

304. Sjostrom S, Tamsen A, Hartvig P, Folkesson R, Terenius L: Cerebrospinal fluid concentrations of substance P and [met]enkephalin-Arg6-Phe7 during surgery and patient-controlled analgesia. *Anesth Analg* 67: 976-981, 1988.

305. Nyberg F, Liu Z, Lind C, Thornwall M, Ordeberg G: Enhanced CSF levels of substance P in patients with painful arthrosis but not in patients with pain from herniated lumbar discs. [Abstract] *J Musculoske Pain* 3 (Suppl 1):2, 1995.

306. Russell IJ: [Unpublished]

307. Vaeroy H, Nyberg F, Terenius L: No evidence for endorphin deficiency in fibromyalgia following investigation of cerebrospinal fluid [CSF] dynorphin A and Met–enkephalin-Arg6-Phe7. *Pain* 46:139-143, 1991.

308. Giovengo SL, Russell IJ, Larson AA: Increased concentrations of nerve growth factor in cerebrospinal fluid of patients with fibromyalgia. *J Rheumatol* 26: 1564-1569, 1999.

309. Russell IJ: [Unpublished]

310. Vanderah TW, Laughlin T, Lashbrook JM, Nichols ML, Wilcox GL, Ossipov MH: Single intrathecal injections of dynorphin A or des-tyr-dynorphins produce long-lasting allodynia in rats: blockade by MK-801 but not naloxone. *Pain* 68:275-281, 1996.

311. Smullin DH, Skilling SR, Larson AA: Interactions between substance P, calcitonin gene-related peptide, taurine and excitatory amino acids in the spinal cord. *Pain* 42:93-101, 1990.

312. Okano K, Kuraishi Y, Satoh M: Involvement of substance P and excitatory amino acids in aversive behavior elicited by intrathecal capsaicin. *Neurosci Res* 19:125-130, 1994.

313. Larson AA, Giovengo SL, Russell IJ, Michalek JE: Changes in the concentrations of amino acids in the cerebrospinal fluid that correlate with pain in patients with fibromyalgia: implications for nitric oxide pathways. *Pain* 87(2):201-211, 2000.

314. King AE, Lopez-Garcia JA: Excitatory amino acid receptor-mediated neurotransmission from cutaneous afferents in rat dorsal horn in vitro. *J Physiol* 472: 443-457, 1993.

315. Aanonsen LM, Lei S, Wilcox GL: Excitatory amino acid receptors and nociceptive neurotransmission in rat spinal cord. *Pain* 41:309-321, 1990.

316. Cotman CW, Iversen LL: Excitatory amino acids in the brain–focus on NMDA receptors. *TINS* 10:263-265, 1987.

317. Westlund KN, McNeill DL, Coggeshall RE: Glutamate immunoreactivity in rat dorsal root axons. *Neurosci Lett* 96:13-17, 1998.

318. Okano K, Kuraishi Y, Satoh M: Pharmacological evidence for involvement of excitatory amino acids in aversive responses induced by intrathecal substance P in rats. *Biol Pharm Bull* 16:861-865, 1993.

319. Aanonsen LM, Wilcox GL: Nociceptive action of excitatory amino acids in the mouse; effects of spinally administered opioids, phencyclidine and sigma agonists. *J Pharmacol Exp Ther* 243:9-19, 1987.

320. Sorkin LS, McAdoo DJ, Willis WD: Raphe magnus stimulation-induced antinociception in the cat is associated with release of amino acids as well as serotonin in the lumbar dorsal horn. *Brain Res* 618:95-108, 1993.

321. Panter SS, Yum SW, Faden AI: Alteration in extracellular amino acids after traumatic spinal cord injury. [See comments] *Ann Neurol* 27:96-99, 1990.

322. Long JB, Rigamonti DD, Oleshansky MA, Wingfield CP, Martinez-Arizala A: Dynorphin A-induced rat spinal cord injury: evidence for excitatory amino acid involvement in a pharmacological model of ischemic spinal cord injury. *J Pharm Exper Therapeut* 269:358-366, 1994.

323. Mao J, Price DD, Hayes RL, Lu J, Mayer DJ: Differential roles of NMDA and non-NMDA receptor activation in induction and maintenance of thermal hyperalgesia in rats with painful peripheral mononeuropathy. *Brain Res* 598:271-278, 1992.

324. Miller BA, Woolf CJ: Glutamate-mediated slow synaptic currents in neonatal rat deep dorsal horn neurons in vitro. *J Neurophysiol* 76:1465-1476, 1996.

325. Oye I, Rabben T, Fagerlund TH: [Analgesic effect of ketamine in a patient with neuropathic pain.] [Norwegian] *Tidsskrift for Den Norske Laegeforening* 116:3130-3131, 1996.

326. Nyberg F, LeGreves P, Sundqvist C, Terenius L: Characterization of substance P(1-7) and (1-8) generating enzyme in human cerebrospinal fluid. *Biochem Biophys Res Commun* 125:244-250, 1984.

327. Skilling SR, Smullin DH, Larson AA: Differential effects of C- and N-terminal substance P metabolites on the release of amino acid neurotransmitters from the spinal cord: potential role in nociception. *J Neurosci* 10:1309-1318, 1990.

328. Yukhananov RYU, Larson AA: An N-terminal fragment of substance P, substance P(1-7), down-regulates neurokinin-1 binding in the mouse spinal cord. *Neurosci Lett* 178:163-166, 1994.

329. Moldofsky H, Warsh JJ: Plasma tryptophan and musculoskeletal pain in nonarticular rheumatism ["fibrositis syndrome"]. *Pain* 5:65-71, 1978.

330. Yunus MB, Dailey JW, Aldag JC, Masi AT, Jobe PC: Plasma tryptophan and other amino acids in primary fibromyalgia: a controlled study. *J Rheumatol* 19(1): 90-94, 1992.

331. Russell IJ, Michalek JE, Vipraio GA, Fletcher EM, Wall K: Serum amino acids in fibrositis/fibromyalgia syndrome. *J Rheumatol*, Supplement 19:158-163, 1989.

332. Russell IJ, Vipraio GA, Acworth I: Abnormalities in the central nervous system [CNS] metabolism of tryptophan [TRY] to 3-hydroxy kynurenine [OHKY] in fibromyalgia syndrome [FS]. *Arthritis Rheum* 36(9): S222, 1993.

333. Russell IJ, Michalek JE, Vipraio GA, Fletcher EM, Javors MA, Bowden CA: Platelet 3H-imipramine uptake receptor density and serum serotonin levels in patients with fibromyalgia/fibrositis syndrome. *J Rheumatol* 19:104-109, 1992.

334. Hrycaj P, Stratz T, Muller W: Platelet 3H-imipramine uptake receptor density and serum serotonin in patients with fibromyalgia/fibrositis syndrome. *J Rheumatol* 20:1986-1987, 1993.

335. Russell IJ, Vipraio GA: Serotonin [5HT] in serum and platelets [PLT] from fibromyalgia patients [FS]

and normal controls [NC]. *Arthritis Rheum* 37(Suppl): S214, 1994.

336. Russell IJ, Vaeroy H, Javors M, Nyberg F: Cerebrospinal fluid biogenic amine metabolites in fibromyalgia/fibrositis syndrome and rheumatoid arthritis. *Arthritis Rheum* 35:550-556, 1992.

337. Klein R, Bansch M, Berg PA: Clinical relevance of antibodies against serotonin and gangliosides in patients with primary fibromyalgia syndrome. *Psycho-Neuro-Endocrinol* 17:593-598, 1992.

338. Vedder CI, Bennett RM: An analysis of antibodies to serotonin receptors in fibromyalgia. *J Musculoske Pain*; 3(Suppl 1):73, 1995.

339. Russell IJ: [Unpublished]

340. Wolfe F, Ross K, Anderson J, Russell IJ, Hebert L: The prevalence and characteristics of fibromyalgia in the general population. *Arthritis Rheum* 38:19-28, 1995.

341. Nishizawa S, Benkelfat C, Young SN, Leyton M, Mzengeza S, DeMontigny C, Blier P, Diksic M: Differences between males and females in rates of serotonin synthesis in human brain. *Proc Natl Acad Sci USA* 94:5308-5313, 1997.

342. Culman J, Unger T: Central tachykinins: mediators of defense reaction and stress reactions. [Review] [54 refs] *Can J Physiol Pharm* 73:885-891, 1995.

343. Velazquez RA, Kitto KF, Larson AA: CP-96, 345, which inhibits [3H] substance P binding, selectively inhibits the behavioral response to intrathecally administered N-methyl-D-aspartate, but not substance P, in the mouse. *J Pharm Experiment Therapeut* 281: 1231-1237, 1997.

344. Yashpal K, Radhakrishnan V, Henry JL: NMDA receptor antagonist blocks the facilitation of the tail flick reflex in the rat induced by intrathecal administration of substance P and by noxious cutaneous stimulation. *Neurosci Lett* 128:269-272, 1991.

345. Raigorodsky G, Urca G: Involvement of NMDA receptors in nociception and motor control in the spinal cord of the mouse: behavioral, pharmacological and electrophysiological evidence. *Neurosci* 36:601-610, 1990.

346. Ren K, Dubner R: NMDA receptor antagonists attenuate mechanical hyperalgesia in rats with unilateral inflammation of the hind paw. *Neurosci Lett* 163:22-26, 1993.

347. Littman BH, Newton FA, Russell IJ: Substance P antagonism in fibromyalgia: a trial with CJ-11,974. *Pain* (Suppl), 1999.

348. McCain GA, Tibe KS: Diurnal hormone variation in fibromyalgia syndrome: a comparison with rheumatoid arthritis. *J Rheumatol* 19(Suppl):154-157, 1989.

349. Ferraccioli G, Cavalieri F, Salaffi F, Fontana S, Scita F, Nolli M, Maestri D: Neuroendocrinologic findings in primary fibromyalgia and in other chronic rheumatic conditions. *J Rheumatol* 17:869-873, 1990.

350. Griep EN, Boersma JW, deKloet ER: Evidence for neuroendocrine disturbance following physical exercise in primary fibromyalgia syndrome. *J Musculoske Pain* 1(3,4):217-222, 1993.

351. Adler JE, Nauth K, Mossey CJ, Gleason R, Komaroff A, Goldenberg DL: Reduced pituitary and adrenal responses to hypoglycemia in women with fibromyalgia syndrome. *Arthritis Rheum* 39(Suppl 9):S276, 1996.

352. Lentjes EG, Griep EN, Boersma JW, Romijn FP, De Kloet ER: Glucocorticoid receptors, fibromyalgia and low back pain. *Psychoneuroendocrinol* 22:603-614, 1997.

353. Bennett RM, Clark SR, Walczyk J: A randomized, double blind, placebo-controlled study of growth hormone in the treatment of fibromyalgia. *Am J Med* 104:227-231, 1998.

354. Bennett RM, Cook DM, Clark SR, Burckhardt CS, Campbell SM: Hypothalamic-pituitary-insulin-like growth factor-1 axis dysfunction in patients with fibromyalgia. *J Rheumatol* 24:1384-1389, 1997.

355. Clauw DJ, Radulovic D, Heshmat Y, Barbey JT: Heart rate variability as a measure of autonomic function in patients with fibromyalgia [FM] and chronic fatigue syndrome [CFS]. *J Musculoske Pain* 3(Suppl 1): 78, 1995.

356. Clauw DJ, Chrousos GP: Chronic pain and fatigue syndromes: overlapping clinical and neuroendocrine features and potential pathogenic mechanisms. *Neuroimmunomodulation* 4:134-153, 1997.

357. Bou-Holaigah I, Calkins H, Flynn JA, Tunin C, Chang HC, Kan JS, Rowe PC: Provocation of hypotension and pain during upright tilt table testing in adults with fibromyalgia. *Clin Exper Rheumatol* 15:239-246, 1997.

358. Rowe PC, Bou-Holaigah I, Kan JS, Calkins H: Is neurally mediated hypotension an unrecognized cause of chronic fatigue? *Lancet* 345:623-624, 1995.

359. Armario A, Marti O, Gavalda A: Negative feedback of corticosterone on the pituitary-adrenal axis is maintained after inhibition of serotonin synthesis with parachlorophenylalanine. *Brain Res Bull* 28:915-918, 1992.

360. Gartside SE, Cowen PH: Mediation of ACTH and prolactin responses to 5-HTP by 5-HT2 receptors. *Euro J Pharmacol* 179:103-109, 1990.

361. Coiro V, Volpi R, Capretti L, Speroni G, Bianconi L, Cavazzini U: 5-HT1-, but not 5-HT2-serotonergic, M1-, M2-muscarinic cholinergic or dopaminergic receptors mediate the ACTH/cortisol response to metoclopramide in man. *Horm Resear* 33:233-238, 1990.

362. Lesch KP, Sohnle K, Poten B, Schoellnhammer G, Rupprecht R, Schulte HM: Corticotropin and cortisol secretion after central 5-hydroxytryptamine-1A [5-HT1A] receptor activation: effects of 5-HT receptor and beta-adrenoceptor antagonists. *J Clin Endocrinol Metabol* 70:670-674, 1990.

363. King BH, Brazell C, Dourish CT, Middlemiss DN: MK-212 increases rat plasma ACTH concentration by activation of the 5-HT1C receptor subtype. *Neurosci Lett* 105:174-176, 1989.

364. Fuller RW: Serotonin receptors and neuroendocrine responses. *Neuropsychophamacol* 3:495-502, 1990.

365. Feldman S: Neural pathways mediating adrenocortical responses. *Fed Proc Fed Am Soc Exp Biol* 44:169-175, 1985.

366. Przegalinski E, Budziszewska B, Grochmal A: Oxaprotiline enantiomers stimulate ACTH and corticosterone secretion in the rat. *J Neural Transmiss–Gener Sect* 85:211-222, 1991.

367. Torpy DJ, Papanicolaou DA, Lotsikas AJ, Wilder RL, Chrousos GP, Pillemer SR: Responses of the sympathetic nervous system and the hypothalamic-pituitary-adrenal axis to interleukin-6: a pilot study in fibromyalgia. *Arthritis Rheum* 43:872-880, 2000.

368. Maes M, Libbrecht I, Van Hunsel F, Lin AH, De Clerck L, Stevens W: The immune/inflammatory pathophysiology of fibromyalgia: increased serum soluble gp-130, the common signal transducer protein with various neurotropic cytokines. *Psychoneuroendocrinol* 24: 371-383, 1999.

369. Wallace DJ, Bowman RL, Wormsley SB, Peter JB: Cytokines and immune regulation in patients with fibrositis. [published erratum appears in *Arthritis Rheum* 1989 Dec;32(12):1607]. *Arthritis Rheum* 32:1334-1335, 1989.

370. Wallace DJ, Linker-Israeli M, Hallegua D, Silverman S, Silver D, Weisman MH: Do cytokines play a pathogenic role in fibromyalgia?: a hypothesis and pilot study. [Abstract] *J Musculoske Pain* [submitted for MYOPAIN '01, Portland, OR, Sept 9-13, 2001]:2001.

371. Clark S, Tindall E, Bennett RM: A double blind crossover trial of prednisone versus placebo in the treatment of fibrositis. *J Rheumatol* 12:980-983, 1985.

372. Carette S, Dessureault M, Belanger A: Fibromyalgia and sex hormones. *J Rheumatol* 19: 831, 1992.

373. Hapidou EG, Rollman GB: Menstrual cycle modulation of tender points. *Pain* 77:151-161, 1998.

374. Anderberg UM, Marteinsdottir I, Hallman J, Backstrom T: Variability in cyclicity affects pain and other symptoms in female fibromyalgia syndrome patients. *J Musculoske Pain* 6(4):5-22, 1998.

375. Bennett RM, Clark SR, Burckhardt CS, Cook D: IGF-1 assays and other GH tests in 500 fibromyalgia patients. *J Musculoske Pain* 3(Suppl 1):109, 1995.

376. Trommer PR: Hypothyroidism with presenting symptoms of fibrositis. *J Rheumatol* 9:335-336, 1982.

377. Wilke WS, Sheeler LR, Makarowski WS: Hypothyroidism with presenting symptoms of fibrositis. *J Rheumatol* 8:626-631, 1981.

378. Kales A, Heuser G, Jacobson A, Kales JD, Hanley J, Zweizig JR, Paulson MY: All night sleep studies in hypothyroid patients, before and after treatment. *J Clin Endocrinol* 27:1593-1599, 1967.

379. Carette S, Lefrancois L: Fibrositis and primary hypothyroidism. *J Rheumatol* 15:1418-1421, 1988.

380. Lowe JC, Cullum ME, Graf LHJ, Yellin J: Mutations in the c-erbA beta 1 gene: do they underlie euthyroid fibromyalgia? *Med Hypoth* 48:125-135, 1997.

381. Bou-Holaigah I, Rowe PC, Kan J, Calkins H: The relationship between neurally mediated hypotension and the chronic fatigue syndrome. *JAMA* 274:961-967, 1995.

382. Rowe PC, Calkins H: Neurally mediated hypotension and chronic fatigue syndrome. *Am J Med* 104 (3A):15S-21S, 1998.

383. Davies R, Slater JDH, Forsling ML, Payne N: The response of arginine vasopressin and plasma renin to postural change in normal man, with observations of syncope. *Clin Sci* 51:267-274, 1976.

384. Cohen H, Neumann L, Shore M, Amir M, Cassuto Y, Buskila D: Autonomic dysfunction in patients with fibromyalgia: application of power spectral analysis of heart rate variability. *Semin Arthritis Rheum* 29(4): 217-227, 2000.

385. Simpson LO: Nondiscocytic erythrocytes in myalgic encephalomyelitis. *N Z Med J* 102(864):126-127, 1989.

386. Simpson LO: Explanatory notes about red cell shape analysis. Personal communication.

387. Mountz JM, Bradley LA, Modell JG, Alexander RW, Triana-Alexander M, Aaron LS: Fibromyalgia in women. Abnormalities of regional cerebral blood flow in the thalamus and the caudate nucleus are associated with low pain threshold levels. *Arthritis Rheum* 38: 926-938, 1995.

388. Kwiatek R, Barnden L, Tedman R, Jarrett R, Chew J, Rowe C, Pile K: Regional cerebral blood flow in fibromyalgia: single photon-emission computed tomography evidence of reduction in the pontine tegmentum and thalami. *Arthritis Rheum* 43:2823-2833, 2000.

389. Mountz JM, Bradley LA, Alarcon GS: Abnormal functional activity of the central nervous system in fibromyalgia syndrome. *Amer J Med Sci* 315:385-396, 1998.

390. Iadarola MJ, Max MB, Berman KF, Byas-Smith MG, Coghill RC, Gracely RH, Bennett GJ: Unilateral decrease in thalamic activity observed with positron emission tomography in patients with chronic neuropathic pain. *Pain* 63:55-64, 1995.

391. Donaldson M, Donaldson CCS, Mueller HH, Sella G: qEEG pattern, psychological status and pain report for fibromyalgia sufferers. *Amer J Pain Manag* 2003 [in press].

392. Koerber Rk, Torkelson R, Haven G, Donaldson J, Cohen S, Case M: Increased cerebrospinal fluid 5-HT and 5-HIAA in Kliene-Levein syndrome. *Neurol* 34(12): 1597-1600, 1984.

393. Mueller HH, Donaldson CCS, Nelson DV, Layman M: Treatment of fibromyalgia incorporating EEG-driven stimulation: a clinical outcomes study. *J Clin Psychol* 57:933-952, 2001.

394. Donaldson CCS, Snelling LS, MacInnis AL, Sella GE, Mueller HH: Diffuse muscular coactivation [DMC] as a potential source of pain in fibromyalgia–part 1. *J Neurorehab* 17(1):33-39, Feb 2002.

395. Donaldson CCS, MacInnis AL, Snelling LS, Sella GE, Mueller HH: Characteristics of diffuse muscular coactivation [DMC] in fibromyalgia sufferers–part 2. *J Neurorehab* 17(1):41-48, Feb 2002.

396. Rosner MJ, Guin SE, Johnson A, Rosner SE: Craniocervical decompression, cerebral blood flow, and neuropsychological dysfunction in FMS and CFS. *National Fibromyalgia Research Foundation Conference*, Portland, Oregon Sept 26-27, 1999.

397. Heffez DS, Ross RE, Shade-Zeldow Y, Kostas K, Shah S, Gottschalk R, Elias DA, Shepard A, Leurgans SE, Moore CG: Is cervical myelopathy overlooked in patients with fibromyalgia? Presented at the *European Section of the Cervical Spine Research Society*, Paris, France, June 12-15, 2002.

398. Heffez DS, Ross RE, Shade-Zeldow Y, Kostas K, Shah S, Gottschalk R, Elias DA, Shepard A, Leurgans SE, Moore CG: Is there an association between cervical myelopathy and fibromyalgia? Presented at the *European Section of the Cervical Spine Research Society*, Paris, France, June 12-15, 2002.

399. Alarcon GS, Bradley LA, Hadley MN, Sotolongo A, Alberts KR, Martin MY: Does Chiari formation contribute to fibromyalgia [FM] symptoms? *Arthritis Rheum* 40(Suppl 9):S190, 1997.

400. Gracely RH, Petzke F, Wolf JM, Clauw DJ: Functional magnetic resonance imaging evidence of augmented pain processing in fibromyalgia. *Arthritis Rheum* 46(5):1333-1343, 2002.

401. Russell IJ: Unpublished.

402. Staud R, Vierck CJ, Cannon RL, Mauderli AP, Price DD: Abnormal sensitization and temporal summation of second pain [wind-up] in patients with fibromyalgia syndrome. *Pain* 91:165-175, 2001.

403. Russell IJ: Is it my fibromyalgia, doctor? *J Musculoske Pain* 9:1-5, 2001.

404. Cetin A, Sivri A: Respiratory function and dyspnea in fibromyalgia syndrome. *J Musculoske Pain* 9(1):7-16, 2001.

405. Mengshoel AM, Forre O, Komnaes HB: Muscle strength and aerobic capacity in primary fibromyalgia. *Clin Exp Rheumatol* 8:475-479, 1990.

406. Lurie M, Caidahl K, Johansson G, Bake B: Respiratory function in chronic primary fibromyalgia. *Scand J Rehabil Med* 22:151-155, 1990.

407. Yunus MB, Masi AT, Aldag JC: A controlled study of primary fibromyalgia syndrome: clinical features and association with other functional syndromes. *J Rheumatol* 19:62-71, 1989.

408. Triadafilopoulos G, Simms RW, Goldenberg DL: Bowel dysfunction in fibromyalgia syndrome. *Digest Dis Sci* 36:59-64, 1991.

409. Romano TJ: Coexistence of irritable bowel syndrome and fibromyalgia. *WV Med J* 84:16-18, 1988.

410. Murthy SN, DePace DM, Shah RS, Podell R: Acute effect of substance P in immunologic vasculitis in the rat colon. *Peptides* 12:1337-1345, 1991.

411. Buskila D, Odes LR, Neumann L, Odes HS: Fibromyalgia in inflammatory bowel disease. *J Rheumatol* 26:1167-1171, 1999.

412. Palm O, Moum B, Jahnsen J, Gran JT: Fibromyalgia and chronic widespread pain in patients with inflammatory bowel disease: a cross sectional population survey. *J Rheumatol* 28:590-594, 2001.

413. Gladman DF, Urowitz MB, Gough J, MacKinnon A: Fibromyalgia as a major contributor of quality of life and lupus. *J Rheumatol* 24:2145-2148, 1997.

414. Hester G, Grant AE, Russell IJ: Psychological evaluation and behavioral treatments with fibrositis. [Abstract] *Arthritis Rheum* 25:S148, 1982.

415. Leavitt F, Katz RS, Golden HE, Glickman PB, Layfer LF: Comparison of pain properties in fibromyalgia patients and rheumatoid arthritis patients. *Arthritis Rheum* 29:775, 1986.

416. Dohrenbusch R, Gruterich R, Genth M: Fibromyalgia and Sjögren's Syndrome: clinical and methodological aspects. *Z Rheumatol* 55:19-27, 1996.

417. Alagiri M, Chottiner S, Ratner V, Slade D, Hanno PM: Interstitial cystitis: unexplained association with other chronic disease and pain syndromes. *Urology* 49:52-57, 1997.

418. Bennett R: Fibromyalgia, chronic fatigue syndrome, and myofascial pain. *Curr Opin Rheum* 10:95-103, 1998.

419. Clauw DJ, Schmidt M, Radulovic D, Singer A, Katz P, Bresette J: The relationship between fibromyalgia and interstitial cystitis. *J Psychia Res* 31:125-131, 1997.

420. Wieling W, van Lieshout JJ, van Leeuwen AM: Physical maneuvers that reduce postural hypotension in autonomic failure. *Clin Autonom Res* 3:57-65, 1993.

421. Van Lieshout JJ, Ten Harkel ADJ, Wieling W: Physical maneuvers for combating orthostatic dizziness in autonomic failure. *Lancet* 339:897-898, 1992.

422. Walther DS: Applied Kinesiology. *Systems DC*, Colorado 1976.

423. Corning P: Inaccurate evaluations used to assess individuals with ME/CFS. *Quest* 2000 Dec/Jan; 39. *http://www.mefmaction.net* [Information regarding CSA Actigraph can be obtained from *http://csainc.net*]

424. van der Werf SP, Prins JB, Vercoulen JH, van der Mer JW, Bleijenberg G: Identifying physical activity patterns in chronic fatigue syndrome using actigraphic assessment. *J Psychosom Res* 49(5):373-379, 2000.

425. Henriksson CM, Gundmark I, Bengtsson A, Ek AC: Living with fibromyalgia. Consequences for everyday life. *Clin J Pain* 8:138-144, 1992.

426. Hawley DJ, Wolfe F: Pain, disability and pain/disability relationships in seven rheumatic disorders: a study of 1,522 patients. *J Rheumatol* 18:1552-1557, 1991.

427. Henriksson CM: Living with continuous muscular pain–patient perspectives. Part I: Encounters and consequences. *Scand J Caring Sci* 9:67-76, 1995.

428. Bennett RM: Fibromyalgia and the disability dilemma. A new era in understanding a complex multidimensional pain syndrome. *Arthritis Rheum* 39:1627-1634, 1996.

429. Waylonis GW, Ronan PG, Gordon C: A profile of fibromyalgia in occupational environments. *Am J Phys Med Rehabil* 73:112-115, 1994.

430. King PM, Tuckwell N, Barrett TE: A critical review of Functional Capacity Evaluation. *Physical Ther* 78:852-866, 1998.

431. Olin RJ: Neuroendocrinological Syndromes: a new paradigm with important consequences for the patient, the medical community and research. Guest of Honor Lecturer, *5th Annual Fibromyalgia and Chronic Fatigue International Conference*, Seattle, Washington, Feb. 2-5, 1996.

432. Smythe H: Problems with the MMPI. *J Rheumatol* 11:4, 1984.

433. Main CJ, Waddell G: Behavioral responses to examination: A reappraisal of the interpretation of "non-organic signs." *Spine* 23(21):2367-2371, 1998.

APPENDICES

1. GLOSSARY OF ACRONYMS

2. SYMPTOMS AND SIGNS

3. FMS CLINICAL DIAGNOSTIC WORKSHEET

4. MYOFASCIAL PAIN SYNDROME

5. DIFFERENTIAL DIAGNOSIS OF FMS SYMPTOMS

6. SYMPTOM SEVERITY AND HIERARCHY PROFILE [SSHP]

7. PAIN VISUAL ANALOG SCALE [PAIN VAS], BODY PAIN DIAGRAM

8. SLEEP PROFILE [SP]

9. FIBROMYALGIA IMPACT QUESTIONNAIRE [FIQ]

10. INSTRUCTIONS FOR MRI

11. HOW TO DO N = 1 TRIALS

12. BODY TEMPERATURE

13. DIZZINESS AND NEURALLY MEDIATED HYPOTENSION

14. PROPER BODY MECHANICS AND ERGONOMICS

15. RELAXATION TECHNIQUES

16. SELF-POWERED STRETCHES AND EXERCISES FOR FMS PATIENTS

17. ASSESSING OCCUPATIONAL DISABILTY

18. WORK PLACE AGGRAVATORS

19. TESTS THAT MAY BE USED INAPPROPRIATELY FOR FMS

20. AUTHORS' AFFILIATIONS AND ACKNOWLEDGMENTS

APPENDIX 1. Glossary of Acronyms

ACR:	American College of Rheumatology
ACTH:	adrenocorticotropin hormone
ANS:	autonomic nervous system
BBB:	blood brain barrier
CFS:	chronic fatigue syndrome
CGRP:	calcitonin gene-related peptide
CNS:	central nervous system
COX2:	cyclooxygenase-2
CRF:	corticotrophin releasing factor
CSF:	cerebrospinal fluid
CT:	computed tomography
CTS:	carpal tunnel syndrome
DHEA:	dehydroepiandrosterone
DSM:	diagnostic and statistical manual
EAAs:	excitatory amino acids
EEG:	electroencephalogram
qEEG:	quantitative electroencephalogram
EEG-S:	electroencephalographic spectrum
FM:	fibromyalgia [not the best abbreviation or term]
FMS:	fibromyalgia syndrome
GABA:	gammaaminobutyric acid
GI:	gastrointestinal
GU:	genitourinary
HA:	hyaluronic acid
HGH:	human growth hormone
5-HHIA:	5-hydroxyindoleacetic acid
HLA:	human leukocyte antigens
HNC:	healthy normal controls
HPA:	hypothalamic-pituitary-adrenal
HPG:	hypothalamic-pituitary-gonadal
HPGH:	hypothalamic-pituitary-growth hormone
HPT:	hypothalamic-pituitary-thyroid
HRT:	hormone replacement therapy
5-HTP:	5-hydroxytryptophan
IGF1:	insulin-like growth factor–1
IMS:	intramuscular stimulation
kDa:	kilodalton
LE:	level of evidence
MAO:	monoamine oxidase
ME:	myalgic encephalomyelitis
ME/CFS:	myalgic encephalomyelitis/chronic fatigue syndrome
MPS:	myofascial pain syndrome

MRI:	magnetic resonance imaging
fMRI:	functional magnetic resonance imaging
NGF:	nerve growth factor
NK1:	neurokinin-1
NMDA:	N-methyl-D-asparate
NMH:	neurally mediated hypotension
NMR:	nuclear magnetic resonance
NO:	nitric oxide
NSAID:	nonsteroidal anti-inflammatories
OA:	osteoarthritis
OT:	occupational therapist
PCO:	procyanidolic oligomers
PET:	positron emission tomography
PFC:	prefrontal cortex
PFMS:	primary fibromyalgia syndrome
RA:	rheumatoid arthritis
RBC:	red blood cell
rCBF:	regional cerebral blood flow
RCT:	randomized control trial
REM:	rapid eye movements
RNAse L:	ribonuclease L
SAD:	seasonal affective disorder
SCM:	sternocleidomastoid muscles
SEA Tech:	synaptic electronic activation technology
SFMS:	secondary fibromyalgia syndrome, FMS associated with other conditions
SLE:	systemic lupus erythematosus
SNRI:	serotonin noradrenergic reuptake inhibitor
SP:	substance P
SPECT:	single-photon emission computed tomography
SSRI:	selective serotonin reuptake inhibitor
T3:	triiodothyronine
T4:	tetraiodothyronine
TENS:	transcutaneous electrical nerve stimulation
TePs:	tender points
TMJ:	temporomandibular joint
TPI:	tender point index
TRH:	thyrotropin-releasing hormone
TRP:	tryptophan
TrPs:	trigger points
TSH:	thyroid-stimulating hormone

APPENDIX 2. Symptoms and Signs

As the neurological and endocrine systems are widely distributed, symptoms are numerous, multiform and of variable intensities. Many of the following symptoms and signs are not present in everyone or at all times and, therefore, cannot be included as part of the criteria for diagnosis.

Musculoskeletal System
- generalized stiffness 80 percent
- muscle cramps–e.g., legs 40 percent
- chest pressure and pain
- TMJ

Nervous System
- persistent fatigue 87 percent
- lack of endurance 67 percent
- migraines or new onset headaches 58 percent

Sensory
- hypersensitivity to pain
- hyper-responsiveness to noxious stimuli
- perceptual and dimensional distortions
- feeling of burning or swelling
- sensory overload phenomena
- loss of cognitive map
- dyspnea

Cognitive
- difficulties processing information
- slowness in cognitive processing
- concentration problems
- difficulties with word retrieval
- confusion and word mix-ups
- short-term memory difficulties

Motor and Balance
- muscle weakness and paralysis
- poor balance, ataxia and tandem gait
- clumsiness and tendency to drop things
- difficulty in tandem gait
- atypical numbness or tingling 64 percent

Neuroendocrine System
- marked weight change
- heat/cold intolerance 85 percent
- neuropsychological
- mood swings, anxiety 60 percent
- reactive depression

Visual and Auditory Disturbances
- visual changes or eye pain
- double, blurred or wavy vision
- dry or itchy eyes
- photophobia
- tinnitus–buzzing or ringing in ears
- hyperacusis and interference from background noise

Sleep Disturbances 82 percent
- sleep disorders–hyper or insomnia
- non-refreshing sleep

Circulatory System
- neurally mediated hypotension
- fainting or vertigo
- palpitations and tachycardia
- fluid retention
- bruising

Digestive System
- lump in throat
- nausea
- heart burn
- abdominal pain
- irritable bowel syndrome 40 percent

Urinary System
- irritable bladder
- overactive bladder

Reproductive System
- dysmenorrhea
- PMS or irregular menstrual cycles
- loss of sexual libido or impotence
- anorgasmia

APPENDIX 3. Fibromyalgia Syndrome Clinical Worksheet

NAME _____ **DATE** _____

History of Widespread Pain Lasting at Least 3 Months
_____ pain in both sides of the body, above and below the waist [including low back pain]
_____ axial skeletal pain [cervical spine, anterior chest, thoracic spine or low back]

Pain in at Least 11 of 18 Tender Point Sites on 4 kg Palpation [thumbnail whitens]
_____ **Occiput [2]**–at the suboccipital muscle insertions
_____ **Low Cervical [2]**–at the anterior aspects of the intertransverse spaces at C5-C7
_____ **Trapezius [2]**–midpoint of the upper border
_____ **Supraspinatus [2]**–at origins, above the scapula spine near the medial border
_____ **Second rib [2]**–just lateral to the second costochondral junctions on the upper rib surfaces
_____ **Lateral epicondyles [2]**–2 cm distal to the epicondyles [in the brachioradialis muscle]
_____ **Gluteal [2]**–in upper outer quadrants of buttocks in the anterior fold of muscle
_____ **Greater trochanter [2]**–posterior to the trochanter prominence
_____ **Knee [2]**–at medial fat pad proximal to joint line

Additional Clinical Symptoms & Signs
The clinical diagnosis, in addition to the above pain factors, some of these additional clinical symptoms and signs are present in most FMS patients, and can contribute importantly to the patient's burden of illness.

Neurological Manifestations: Include hypertonic and hypotonic muscles; musculoskeletal asymmetry, dysfunction involving muscles; ligaments and joints; atypical patterns of numbness and tingling; abnormal muscle twitch response, muscle cramps, muscle weakness and fasciculations; headaches, generalized weakness, perceptual disturbances, spatial instability and sensory overload phenomena.

Clinical Neurocognitive Manifestations: Some neurocognitive difficulties usually are present. These include impaired concentration and short-term memory consolidation, impaired speed of performance, and/or inability to multi-task.

Fatigue: There is persistent and reactive fatigue accompanied by reduced physical and mental stamina, which often interferes with the patient's ability to exercise.

Sleep Dysfunction: The patient experiences unrefreshed sleep. This is usually accompanied by sleep disturbances including insomnia, frequent nocturnal awakening, nocturnal myoclonus, and/or restless leg syndrome.

Clinical Autonomic and/or Neuroendocrine Manifestations: These manifestations include cardiac arrhythmias, neurally mediated hypotension, vertigo, vasomotor instability, sicca syndrome, temperature instability, heat/cold intolerance, respiratory disturbances, intestinal and bladder motility disturbances with or without irritable bowel or bladder dysfunction, dysmenorrhea, loss of adaptability and tolerance for stress, emotional flattening, lability and/or reactive depression.

Stiffness: Body or muscular stiffness that is most severe in the morning, and often lasting hours. It can return during periods of inactivity during the day.

The compulsory criteria for pain are adopted from, The American College of Rheumatology 1990 Criteria for the Classification of Fibromyalgia: Report of the Multicenter Criteria Committee. Wolfe F, Smythe HA, Yunus MB, Bennett RM, Bombardier C, Goldenberg DL, Tugwell P, Campbell SM, Abeles M, Clark P, Fam AG, Farber SJ, Fiechtner JJ, Franklin CM, Gatter RA, Hamaty D, Lessard J, Lichtbroun AS, Masi AT, McCain GA, Reynolds WJ, Romano TJ, Russell IJ, Sheon RP. © Arthritis and Rheumatism, 1990 February; 33(2):160-172. Reprinted by permission of Wiley-Liss, Inc., a subsidiary of John Wiley & Sons.

APPENDIX 4. Myofascial Pain Syndrome

Myofascial Pain Syndrome involves the sensory, motor, and autonomic symptoms caused by myofascial trigger points. Many FMS patients also have myofascial trigger points. A myofascial trigger point [TrP] is a hyperirritable locus within a taut band of skeletal muscle, located in muscular tissue and/or its associated fascia. The spot is painful on compression, and can evoke characteristic referred pain and autonomic phenomena. An active trigger point causes dysfunction of the affected muscles with restriction of movement. This has been found to be one of the most common causes of longstanding pain. Trigger points, unless treated properly, may persist for decades and affected muscles respond to work or exercise beyond their limits by becoming more dysfunctional and painful. Normal muscles do not contain trigger points or taut bands of muscle fibers, are not tender to firm palpation, exhibit no local twitch response, and do not refer pain in response to applied pressure.

Recommended Criteria for Identifying
a Latent Trigger Point or an Active Trigger Point*‡

Essential Criteria
1. Taut band palpable [if muscle accessible].
2. Exquisite spot tenderness of a nodule in a taut band.
3. Patient's recognition of current pain complaint by pressure on the tender nodule [identifies an active trigger point].
4. Painful limit to full stretch range of motion.

Confirmatory Observations
1. Visual or tactile identification of local twitch response.
2. Imaging of a local twitch response induced by needle penetration of tender nodule.
3. Pain or altered sensation [in the distribution expected from a trigger point in that muscle] on compression of tender nodule.
4. Electromyographic demonstration of spontaneous electrical activity characteristic of active loci in the tender nodule of a taut band.

* Simons DG, Travell JG, Simons LS. Travell & Simons' Myofascial Pain and Dysfunction: The Trigger Point Manual, Volume 1. Upper Half of Body, Second Edition. Table 2.4B, page 35. ©*Williams & Wilkins, A Waverly Company*, Baltimore 1999.

Reprinted with permission of Dr. D. G. Simons, and Williams & Wilkins, A Waverly Company.

‡ Note that a trigger point, TrP, as desribed for MPS, is a different phenomenon that of a tender point, TeP, as described for FMS.

APPENDIX 5. Differential Diagnosis of Fibromyalgia Syndrome Symptoms

Consider alternate sources or causes for these FMS symptoms so that the patient is not subjected to unnecessary and sometimes potentially harmful investigations and treatments.

Headache: vascular migraine, space-occupying intracranial lesions, temporal arteritis

Ocular disturbance/pain: glaucoma, iritis

Auricular disturbance/pain: otitis interna/media/externa, posterior fossa tumor

Sinonasal pain/stuffiness: infective or vasomotor rhinitis/sinusitis

Temporomandibular pain: temporal arteritis

Neck spasm/swelling: lymphadenopathy

Dysphagia: obstructive lesion, pharyngitis

Dysphonia: laryngitis

Dyspnea: pulmonary disease, airway obstruction

Chest pain: pleurisy, pulmonary embolism, angina pectoris, myocardial infarction, pericarditis, gastroesophageal reflux, costochondritis

Abdominal pain: intraabdominal pathology, renal colic

Irritable bowel: bowel infection/infestation/inflammation, villous adenoma, diverticulitis

Irritable bladder: bladder infection, renal colic

Pelvic pain: pelvic organ pathology

Dizziness/imbalance: vestibular neuronitis, cardiac arrhythmia, cerebellar dysfunction

Swelling/vasomotor instability of extremities: arthritis, impaired circulation

Cognitive impairment: Alzheimer's, depression

Paresthesia/weakness: multiple sclerosis, peripheral neuropathy

Claudication: vascular insufficiency

APPENDIX 6. Symptom Severity and Hierarchy Profile [SSHP]

NAME _____ DATE _____

1. Rank your symptoms in order of severity, with one being your most severe symptom.
2. Rate severity of symptoms by putting a check mark in the appropriate column to the right of symptoms.

SYMPTOM SEVERITY AND HIERARCHY CHART					
RANK	**SYMPTOM**	**ABSENT**	**MILD**	**MODERATE**	**SEVERE**
	Pain: in muscles, joints or headaches				
	Fatigue: persistent marked fatigue that reduces activity level, muscle fatigue				
	Sleep Disturbance: non-restorative sleep, insomnia, or frequent awakenings				
	Cognitive Difficulties: 'brain fog,' difficulty in concentration, poor short-term memory, slow speed of performance				
	Functionality: symptoms interfere with being able to carry out daily activities				

Overall symptom severity: _____ mild, _____ moderate, _____ severe
[**Mild**–occurring at rest, **moderate**–symptoms that occur at rest become severe with effort, unable to work, **severe**–often housebound or bed bound.]

Other troublesome symptoms _____

Which symptoms are constant? _____

Which symptoms come and go? _____

Which symptoms have changed and how? _____

What things aggravate your symptoms? _____

What ways have you found to alleviate symptoms? _____

Describe a recent good experience. _____

Is your body temperature normal? _____ Does it fluctuate? _____

How good is your sleep on a scale of 0-10? [10–good refreshing sleep, 0–no sleep] _____

Do you have stiffness in the morning? _____ no, _____ mild, _____ moderate, _____ severe

If you do have morning stiffness, how long does it usually last? _____

How well are you able to function in your daily living activities on a scale of 1-10? [10–able to do daily activities with ease, 1–unable to do daily activities]_____

How do you feel today on a scale of 1-10? [10–terrific, 1–totally bedridden] _____

How do you feel today compared to one month ago? _____ much better, _____ better, _____ about the same, _____ worse, _____ much worse.

Do you have specific concerns or questions you would like to ask? _____
_____
_____

APPENDIX 7. Pain Visual Anolog Scale [PAIN VAS], Body Pain Diagram

NAME _____ DATE _____

1. Please indicate the amount of pain you have had in the last 48 hours by marking a "/" through the line.

| | 0 | 1 | 2 | 3 | 4 | 5 | 6 | 7 | 8 | 9 | 10 |

No Pain   Excruciating Pain

2. On the following diagrams, please indicate your areas of:
   Aching: ======   Burning Pain: xxxxx   Stabbing Pain: ///////////
   Pins & Needles: ooooo   Other Pain: ppppp   Describe: _____

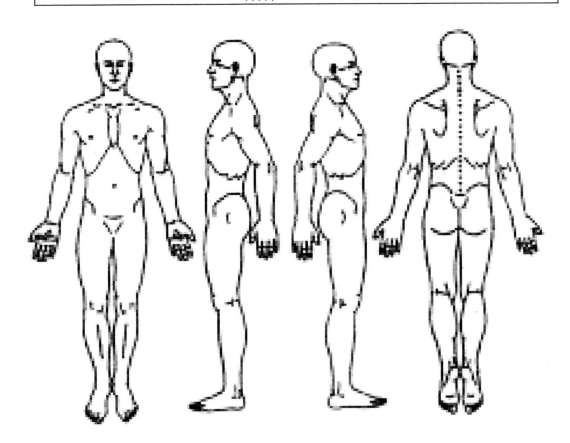

3. How much overall pain relief have you had in the last month?
   Complete [4]   A Lot [3]   Moderate [2]   Slight [1]   None [0]   Worse [−1]

APPENDIX 8. Sleep Profile [SP]

Name _____ **Date** _____ **to** _____

Please complete this chart and for the week prior to your next appointment.

Day	Awakening Time	Temp. a.m.	Time Slept	Sleep Quality	Pain a.m.	Pain p.m.	Temp. p.m.	Bed Time	Min. to Fall Asleep

Temp. a.m.: Take your temperature as soon as you wake up while you are still lying down. Also indicate if you felt cold [C], had cold feet [CF], or cold hands [CH].

Time Slept: Indicate the approximate number of hours and minutes you slept.

Sleep Quality: Good, fair, or poor. Also indicate the number of times you woke during the night including waking up much too early, e.g., if you woke up two times [W2]. Indicate if you know why you woke up–e.g., to urinate, muscle cramps, nasal congestion, etc.

Pain: 0 to 10–0 being no pain, 10 being the worst pain you have experienced.

Temp. p.m.: Take your temperature before going to bed. Indicate if you felt cold.

Min. to Fall Asleep: Indicate approximately how many minutes it took you to fall asleep.

Summary for Week

1. What was your average ~ body temperature when you went to bed? _____
2. What was your average ~ body temperature when you woke up? _____
3. What was the average number of minutes it took to get to sleep? _____
4. What was the average number of times you woke up a night? _____
5. Which of these conditions troubled you at night? _____ **restless leg syndrome,** _____ **muscle cramps,** _____ **muscle pain,** _____ **felt cold,** _____ **woke up to urinate,** _____ **nasal congestion,** _____ **woke up short of breath**
6. What time did you usually wake up in the morning? _____
7. How many hours did you sleep on average? _____
8. Circle how you felt when you woke up? **Energetic   Fine   Tired   Exhausted**
9. Were you stiff when you woke up? _____ If so, for how long? _____
10. Was anything in particular bothering you, e.g., family crisis? _____
11. Indicate you average sleep, pain and energy level on a scale of 0-10, 0 being no sleep, pain or energy, 10 being great sleep, extreme pain, or great energy: _____ **Sleep quality,** _____ **Pain level,** _____ **Energy level**

APPENDIX 9. Fibromyalgia Impact Questionnarie [FIQ]

NAME _____ **DATE** _____

Directions: For the 11 items in question #1, please circle the number that best describes how you did over the past week. If you didn't do an activity before you had fibromyalgia, cross the question out.

1. Were you able to:	Always	Usually	Occasionally	Never
Do shopping?	0	1	2	3
Do laundry with a washer and dryer?	0	1	2	3
Prepare meals?	0	1	2	3
Wash dishes/cooking utensils by hand?	0	1	2	3
Vacuum a rug?	0	1	2	3
Make beds?	0	1	2	3
Walk several blocks?	0	1	2	3
Visit friends or relatives?	0	1	2	3
Do yard work?	0	1	2	3
Drive a car?	0	1	2	3
Climb stairs?	0	1	2	3

2. Of the 7 days in the past week, how many days did you feel good?

   0   1   2   3   4   5   6   7

3. How many days last week did you miss work, including housework, due to fibromyalgia?

   0   1   2   3   4   5   6   7

FIBROMYALGIA IMPACT QUESTIONNAIRE [FIQ]–page 2

Directions: For the remaining items, please indicate by marking a "/" through the line at a point that best indicates how you felt overall for the past week.

1. When you worked, how much did pain or other symptoms of your fibromyalgia interfere with your ability to do
your work, including housework?

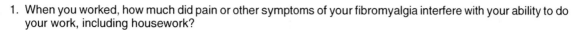

No problem   0   1   2   3   4   5   6   7   8   9   10   Great difficulty
with work   with work

2. How bad has your pain been?

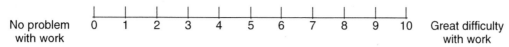

No pain   0   1   2   3   4   5   6   7   8   9   10   Very severe pain

3. How tired have you been?

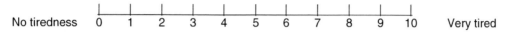

No tiredness   0   1   2   3   4   5   6   7   8   9   10   Very tired

4. How have you felt when you get up in the morning?

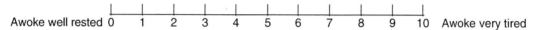

Awoke well rested   0   1   2   3   4   5   6   7   8   9   10   Awoke very tired

5. How bad has your stiffness been?

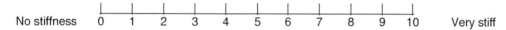

No stiffness   0   1   2   3   4   5   6   7   8   9   10   Very stiff

6. How nervous or anxious have you felt?

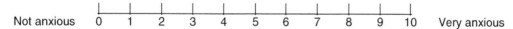

Not anxious   0   1   2   3   4   5   6   7   8   9   10   Very anxious

7. How depressed or blue have you felt?

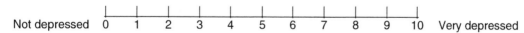

Not depressed   0   1   2   3   4   5   6   7   8   9   10   Very depressed

Reprinted with slight modifications.
Citation: Burckhardt CS, Clark SR, Bennett RM. The Fibromyalgia Impact Questionnaire: Development and Validation. Jour-
nal of Rheumatology 18:728-734, 1991.
Reprinted with permission of Dr. C. S. Burckhardt and the Journal of Rheumatology.

FIBROMYALGIA IMPACT QUESTIONNAIRE [FIQ] SCORING

Purpose: The FIQ is an assessment and evaluation instrument developed to measure fibromyalgia syndrome [FMS] patient status, progress and outcomes. It has been designed to measure the components of health status that are believed to be most affected by FMS. The average FMS patients scores about 50, severely afflicted patients are usually 70 plus.

Content: The FIQ is composed of 20 items. The first 11 items make up a physical functioning scale. Each item is rated on a 4 point likert type scale. Items 12 and 13 ask patients to mark the number of days they felt well and number of days they were unable to work because of FMS symptoms. Items 14 through 20 are visual analog scales marked in 10 increments on which the patient rates work difficulty, pain, fatigue, morning tiredness, stiffness, anxiety and depression.

Scoring: The FIQ is scored in such a way that a higher score indicates a greater impact of fibromyalgia on the person. The maximum possible score is 100. The questionnaire is scored in the following manner:

1. **Question #1 [items 1 through 11]–Physical Impairment:** are scored and summed to yield one physical impairment score. Raw scores on each item can range from 0 [always] to 3 [never]. Because some patients may not do some of the tasks listed, they are given the option of deleting items from scoring. In order to obtain a valid summed score for item 1 through 11, the scores for the items that the patient has rated are summed and divided by the number of items rated. An average raw score between 0 and 3 for question #1 is obtained in this manner.

2. **Question #2 [item 12]–Feel Good:** is reversed so that a higher number indicates impairment [i.e., 0 = 7, 7 = 0, etc.]. Raw scores can range from 0 to 7.

3. **Question #3 [item 13]–Work Missed:** is scored as a number of days the patient was unable to do regular work activities. Raw scores can range from 0 to 7.

4. **Questions #4-10 [items 14 through 20]:** are scored in 10 increments. Raw scores for each question can range from 0 to 10. If the patient marks the space between two numbers, on any item, that item is given a score that includes 0.5.

5. **Normalization Procedure:** Once the initial scoring has been completed, the resulting scores are subjected to a normalization procedure so that all scores are expressed in similar units.
   - Each of the 10 questions has a maximum score of 10–thus scoring of the 0-10 anchored VASs is obvious.
   - You have already given question number 1 [items 1-11] an average score of 0-3. This has to be multiplied by a factor of 3.33 [i.e., $3 \times 3.33 = 10$].
   - The score for question #2 is reversed thus 7 = 0 and 0 = 7. To normalize this score to 10, multiply the score by 1.43.
   - The score for question #3 is also multiplied by 1.43.
   - If one or more questions are missed, multiply the final summative score by 10/x. [i.e., If one question is missed multiply by 10/9 = 1.111, if 2 questions are missed multiply final score by 10/8 = 1.25, etc.].

SCALE	ITEMS	RECODE	SCORE RANGE	NORMALIZATION
1. Physical Impairment	1-11	no	0-3	$S \times 3.33$ [S = raw score]
2. Feel Good	12	yes	0-7	$S \times 1.43$
3. Work Missed	13	no	0-7	$S \times 1.43$
4. Do Job	14	no	0-10	None
5. Pain	15	no	0-10	None
6. Fatigue	16	no	0-10	None
7. Rested	17	No	0-10	None
8. Stiffness	18	No	0-10	None
9. Anxiety	19	No	0-10	None
10. Depression	20	No	0-10	None

Fibromyalgia Impact: The total score provides an estimation of fibromyalgia impact, which ranges from 0 to 100.

Reprinted with slight modifications.
Citation: Burckhardt CS, Clark SR, Bennett RM. The Fibromyalgia Impact Questionnaire: Development and Validation. Journal of Rheumatology 18:728-734, 1991.
Reprinted with permission of Dr. C. S. Burckhardt and the Journal of Rheumatology.

APPENDIX 10. Instructions for MRI

The routine MRI of the cervical spine does not include all of the images necessary for proper evaluation of cervical stenosis. Therefore, clinicians should make an effort to modify the MRI protocol to include: axial cuts oriented parallel to the plane of the foramen magnum, [basion to opisthion] from 2 cm below to 2 cm above the foramen magnum and cervical spine. For evaluation of stenosis, the axial cuts done through each disk should be oriented exactly parallel to the plane of that disk, taking into account that each disk is oriented in a slightly different plane because of the normal curvatures of the neck. This technique avoids artificial enlargement of the canal diameter that occurs if the cut is oblique rather than parallel to the plane of the disk. It is helpful if the ordering doctor view these special axial images him/herself.

The following prevalence of FMS symptoms and neurological signs are based on 270 FMS patients who were referred to a neurosurgeon, Dr. Daniel Heffez, for neurological evaluation. Thus, the prevalence figures may not directly apply to the general FMS population.

FMS symptom [270 patients]	Prevalence percent	Neurological sign	Prevalence percent***
Fatigue**	96	Sensory level*	83
Body pain*	95	Hyper-reflexia**	64
Cognitive impairment	92	Recruitment	57
Generalized weakness*	92	Absent gag reflex	37
Headache*	90	Romberg sign	28
Gait instability*	85	Hoffman sign	26
Grip weakness*	83	Clonus	25
Photophobia	83	Impaired tandem walk	23
Hand clumsiness*	80	Weakness**	22
Paresthesiae*	80	Dysmetria	15
IBS***	77	Impaired position sense	14
Dizziness*	71	Cranial nerve V	8
Numbness *	69	Ataxia	8
Blurred vision/diplopia	65	Nystagmus	6
Disorientation	54	Cranial nerve XII	4
Chronic nausea	40		
* known symptom of myelopathy		* cold and pin stimulus	
** muscular fatigue is a known symptom of myelopathy		** in at least one limb	
*** bowel/bladder dysfunction are associated with myelopathy		*** as determined by the neurosurgeon	

APPENDIX 11. How to Do N = 1 Trials

Prior to and during the trial, have the patient keep other therapies and activities as constant or regular as possible. Instruct patients to keep a symptom diary for two weeks prior to testing and thereafter during trials, marking down good effects, bad effects and side effects. Encourage patients to include standardized, daily sessions of reading or other cognitive activity and physical exercise within fatigue limits and keep a record of the results.

Example: **HYPOTHETICAL PHARMACEUTICAL:** [100-300 mg tid]

Start at 50 mg daily q AM × 3 days
Then 50 mg bid × 4 days
Then 50 mg tid × 7 day
Then 100 mg q AM, 50 mg noon and hs × 3 days
Then 100 mg q AM and noon, and 50 mg hs × 4 days
Then 100 mg tid × 7 days

REASSESS EFFECTIVENESS
Reassess benefits and side effects. Decide whether to discontinue, lower dose, stay at above dose, or increase dose in similar stages to maximum recommended.

WASHOUT PERIOD
There should be a two-week washout between trials.

If it is important to distinguish specific from nonspecific effects for research or other reasons, **and with the patient's permission**, placebo periods can be interspersed.

APPENDIX 12. Body Temperature

It is important to stabilize your body temperature as much as possible.

1. **Normal body temperature is 98.6° Fahrenheit [F] or 37° Celsius [C].**

2. **Your body temperature may be lower than 98.6°F or 37°C.**

3. **Your temperature will go down if:**
   a. You get no sleep
   b. You are in pain or are stiff and sore
   c. You exercise beyond your limits
   d. You do physical work beyond your limits
   e. You are under stress–physical or psychological
   f. You go outside when it is cold
   g. You feel fatigued, ill, etc.

4. **If your temperature is low:**
   a. It will interfere with your sleep
   b. You will be in pain and be stiff
   c. You will be stressed
   d. You will be sensitive to the cold
   e. You will feel fatigued, ill, etc.
   f. You will have problems with exercise and work [weak, tired, etc.]

5. **Your temperature may go up from:**
   a. Eating
   b. Massage therapy
   c. Exercising within your limits
   d. A hot bath or shower

Try to take your temperature when something is happening, e.g., you feel hot or cold, hurt or don't hurt, before and after work or exercise, you feel tired or have more energy, etc. Try to discover things that raise or lower your temperature. You probably will not be able to tell what your temperature is by how you feel.

6. **Bedtime:**
   a. Take your temperature before you go to bed. If it is low or you feel cold, take a hot bath or shower.
   b. Dress warmly. You may need to wear a sweat suit and socks to bed.
   c. Use flannelette sheets on your bed.
   d. Take a hot water bottle to bed or fill a couple 2 liter pop bottles and put them in your bed a half-hour before you go to bed. They will stay warm most of night.

APPENDIX 13. Dizziness and Neurally Mediated Hypotension

A DIZZINESS

Simple instructions to avoid extension or quick rotation of the neck are often sufficient if dizziness is caused by proprioceptive disturbances in the neck.

B. NEURALLY MEDIATED HYPOTENSION [NMH]

1. **Increase salt intake:** Increase salt intake up to 10-15 gm. daily, with an adequate increase in volume of water intake.

2. **Support garments:** Support garments such as support hose and girdles may be helpful.

3. **Physical maneuvers to help alleviate NMH** (382,420,421):
   a. sitting in a knee-chest position
   b. bending forward
   c. when lying down have feet slightly elevated
   d. putting a foot or knee on a chair while standing
   e. squatting

4. **Avoid potential triggers:** The following factors can contribute to early activation of vasovagal reflex and should be avoided.
   a. prolonged standing or sitting
   b. eating large meals
   c. hot showers
   d. hot environments
   e. over-exertion
   f. emotional stress
   g. everyday cognitive stresses
   h. salt depletion
   i. pain

NOTE: Neurally mediated hypotension should be confirmed by tilt table test prior to commencing trials of pharmacological treatments.

APPENDIX 14. Proper Body Mechanics and Ergonomics

Body mechanics refer to the coordinated effort of muscles, bones and the nervous system to maintain proper balance, posture and body alignment. Proper body mechanics allow your body to move and function efficiently with strength and help prevent injury.

A. POSTURE
Proper body alignment helps avoid tired, achy muscles.
  1. Standing
    a. Stand with your feet a comfortable distance apart, approximately shoulder width apart.
    b. Visualize that you have a string attached to the top of your head and someone is holding the string above your head so you can just stand on the ground.
    c. Slightly raise your shoulder until you feel tension, then let them relax so they are square.
    d. Your back should be straight, abdominal muscles tight, lower back flattened and knees relaxed.
    e. Avoid standing for long periods. When you do have to stand, frequently shift position or place one foot on a stool.
  2. Sitting
    a. Choose a firm but comfortable chair with a straight back.
    b. Place lower back against back of chair.
    c. Elbows should always be supported.
    d. Knees should be slightly above hips. Roll a towel under you knees.
    e. Feet should be flat on the floor or stool.
    f. Head should be directly above shoulders.
    g. Avoid sitting forward or with back arched backward.
    h. Take frequent breaks to get up and walk around.
    i. Try not to sit for more than 10-15 minutes at a time.

B. BALANCE
Establish your "center" by the following:[3]
  1. Stand with your feet shoulder width apart.
  2. Gently rock forward until you begin to feel "heavier" or slightly off balance.
  3. Gently rock back until you begin to feel 'heavier.'
  4. Then rock forward until you feel balanced.

C. LIFTING
FMS patients should avoid lifting heavy objects. When you have to do any lifting:
  1. Plan your move and make sure there are no obstacles in your way.
  2. Directly face the object you are lifting to avoid twisting. Turn your whole body if you have to change directions.
  3. Stand in good alignment with your feet shoulder width apart.
  4. Pelvic Tuck: Contract your abdominal muscle and tuck you pelvis forward to help keep your back balanced when lifting. Bend at your knees so you use your largest and strongest muscle groups, which are located in your thighs and hips. Avoid bending from the waist, as that puts maximum strain on the small muscles of the lower back.
  5. Lift and carry load with your shoulders back and your upper arms close to your trunk and your forearms at waist height. Use both hands and arms when lifting. Keep the object close to your body using you large shoulder and upper arm muscles. Avoid holding objects away from your body as that puts strain on the smaller muscles of your lower arms. Stress increases 7 to 10 times when your load is at arm's length.
  6. Use the same techniques for setting the object down.

D. FOOTWEAR
Help avoid tired achy feet by wearing proper footwear.
  1. Shoes should not change the shape of your feet and they should allow freedom to move your toes. They should have arch supports. Shoes should have low heels, which are a maximum of 5 cm [2″] in height, and provide a firm grip for the heel.
  2. Choose shoes made of natural materials that can breathe, e.g., leather and canvas.
  3. It is helpful to use shock-absorbing cushioned insoles.

E. WHEN USING A COMPUTER
[Adapted from information on ergonomics by the Canadian Centre for Occupational Health & Safety [CCOHS][4]]

1. **Desk arrangement:** Place working objects in easy range. Work objects should be able to be seen from a 10-30″ angle below your line of sight.

2. **Chair arrangement:** Use a swivel chair to avoid twisting your body. Adjust the seat to 25-35 cm [10-14″] below the work surface. The back of the chair should give good support and be contoured vertically and horizontally.

3. **Sitting:** Sit up straight. Keep your hips, knees and ankle joints open slightly [90±120″ angle]. The upper body should be 0-30″ forward of an upright position. Keep your shoulders relaxed and upper arms vertical and close to your body. Keep your wrists in line with arms. Your elbows and forearms should be supported with your shoulders slightly elevated to reduce strain on your neck. Most FMS patients find it most comfortable to have the keyboard slightly lower than the waist. Tuck the chin in to slightly lower line of sight 0-30″. Avoid bending neck down. Change position frequently and get up and move around every 15 minutes.

4. **Eye discomfort:** Place the monitor parallel to overhead lighting [not directly below]. Adjust the brightness and contrast of the monitor so it is most comfortable. Have good general lighting and diffuse overhead lighting. Make sure that any lamp focused on written documents is directed away from the monitor to avoid glare. Every few minutes take a few seconds to look away from the screen and focus on distant objects.

   Palming: Close your eyes and cup your hands over your eyes putting gentle pressure on the top of the cheek bones from the base of both palms. Hold for one minute. Blink several times. This helps reduce eye strain.

NOTES

3. Jones KD, Clark SR. Individualizing the exercise prescription for persons with fibromyalgia. *Rheum Dis Clin NA* 28:1-18, 2002.

4. CCOHS Your Environmental Health and Safety Partner. *http://www.ccohs.ca*
   References: http://www.cyber-nurse.com
              http://www.actoronto.org
              http://www.ovenet.uoguelph.ca
              http://www.ot-solutions.on.ca

APPENDIX 15. Relaxation Techniques

Relaxation training techniques are many and varied in the nature of their content and impact upon physiology. They affect body physiology in a general way, triggering a relaxation response by quieting the sympathetic nervous system, thus encouraging your breathing rate, heart rate, and blood pressure to decrease. They can affect the body in specific ways such as by increasing blood flow to different regions of the body. Relaxation techniques also assist in dealing with stress management and improving your overall sense of well-being. The following few examples represent guidelines only.

A. PRINCIPLES

1. **Healing environment:** Set aside a time when you will not be disturbed. The room should be quiet, free from distractions, and be at a comfortable temperature. Sit in a comfortable position in a comfortable chair and relax. Breathe slowly.
2. **Focus:** All relaxation techniques require you to focus on something such as a word, a picture in you mind, your breathing, or an action.
3. **Passive attitude:** Ignore distractions. When other thoughts enter your mind, simply let them go. You can visualize the thought drifting off in a balloon, or on a bird flying across the sky.
4. **Practice is the key to success:** The more you practice the more skilled and efficient you become and the greater benefits you will receive. Enjoy a deep sense of relaxation; minimize muscle tension, and reduce stress.

B. BREATHING EXERCISES

1. **Diaphragmatic breathing:** This allows your lungs to expand and fill more fully. Close your eyes and put one hand on your chest and the other on your upper abdomen at the level of your belly button or stomach. Each time you inhale try to make your hand on your chest remain still and the hand on your abdomen rise. Try to feel your lower lungs filling up with air completely. When you exhale, your hand over your stomach should fall. Feel the air leave your lungs.
2. **Diaphragmatic breath-counting:** While you are doing the same exercise as above, count "one" as you slowly inhale, "two" as you slowly exhale, "three" as you inhale, "four" as you exhale, and so on. Cut off any thoughts that enter your mind.
3. **Complete breath:** After completing diaphragmatic inhalation as in exercise 1, fill the rest of lungs with air to the top above the first rib, at the front, side and back. Then empty the lungs completely from top to bottom. Do not hold the breath. Do two or three cycles.
4. **Pulse breathing:** While you are taking your pulse, inhale and exhale to the same number of pulse beats. Begin with the number of pulse beats that you can do comfortably. Gradually increase the number of pulse beats per breath. Then gradually increase the length of exhalation compared to inhalation up to a maximum of 2:1 ratio.
5. **Spinal extension breathing:** Sit with your legs crossed. Grasp your knees with your hands and keep your elbows straight. As you inhale, begin to extend your back [arching it backwards slightly]. Keep your shoulder down and back. As you exhale, slowly return to starting position. Repeat five to ten times.
6. **Arms out-stretched (422):** Stand with your feet shoulder width apart. Extend your arms to your sides at approximately shoulder height. Turn your left palm to face upward [to tighten the body and help stretch the muscles] and your right palm faces downward. Breathe deeply in and out through your nose ten times. Repeat with your right palm facing upward.
   Option: If you have difficulty standing or holding your arms up, do the exercise sitting on a couch and resting your arms on the back of the couch.
7. **Spinal stretch (422):** Sit in an upright chair with your thighs parallel to the floor, your lower legs perpendicular to the floor, and your feet about shoulder width apart. Bend forward placing your elbows on the inside of your knees. Place your hands between your feet with the backs of your hands facing each other. Then place your fingers under your inner arches so that your palms are facing towards the outside of each foot and rest your thumb over the top of the foot. Let your spine fully stretch while in this position. Breathe slowly and fully for a maximum of five minutes. Do this in the morning. This will help stretch and loosen the spine, making it easier to stand up straight and walk.

C. VISUALIZATION TECHNIQUES

If your mind races and you have difficulty falling asleep because you can not control your thoughts, cognitive and visualization techniques can be helpful. A few examples:

1. **Photographs:** Choose a photograph or a picture from a magazine that is serene and peaceful. Visualize yourself in the picture. If there are flowers, "smell" them or if there is a brook, "listen" to it. As you become more relaxed, feel your stresses float away to be replaced by feelings of peacefulness and happiness.

2. **Visualize a peaceful scene:** This is basically the same as using a photograph but you use your imagination to visualize a peaceful scene such as mountains, streams, oceans, waterfalls, gardens and landscapes, sunrises, sunsets, snow scenes, a spring day, traveling into space, etc. Follow the instructions in C1.

3. **Memory visualization:** Choose a happy memory such as playing on the beach, a birthday party, getting a pet, or doing something well, etc., and picture it in your mind's eye. Let go of your stress and relive your joy.

4. **Guided imagery:** There are numerous audio tapes of guided imagery.

5. **Rewriting a memory:** Choose a troublesome memory and in your imagination "rewrite" the memory the way that you would have liked it to go.

6. **Cognitive thought processing:** Whenever you feel yourself get upset visualize a red stop sign. This alerts you to stop! Take 10 deep diaphragmatic breaths and relax. [You can't concentrate on your diaphragmatic breathing and the stressor at the same time.]

D. AUTOGENIC TRAINING

Autogenic training, developed by Dr. J. H. Schultz, uses relaxation, autosuggestion and visualization techniques to normalize body processes. It is commonly used in Europe in conjunction with pharmaceutical treatments and surgical procedures.

Technique: Relax while sitting or lying down with eyes closed. Adopt an attitude of passive concentration by imagining you are in mental contact with a certain part of your body. Visually or verbally keep repeating a given formula for one minute with a casual attitude toward the results of the exercise. Examples are:

1. **Body relaxation:** Concentrate on your feet feeling heavy and think, "My feet are heavy, they are relaxed, I am at peace." Repeat the same process for your other body parts, e.g., legs, hands, arms, pelvis, chest, neck, and head.

2. **Body warmth:** Use the same method but think of the body parts being warm. This increases blood flow and relaxes blood vessels.

3. **Heartbeat:** Become aware of your heartbeat, then come in "mental contact" with your heart and instruct it to be "calm and regular." This strengthens the self-regulatory process of your heart.

4. **Breathing:** This is the same as #3, but you become aware of your breathing.

5. **Solar plexus:** As above but think, "My solar plexus is warm, heat rays are warming the depth of my abdomen."

E. PROGRESSIVE RELAXATION EXERCISE

Lie down or sit comfortably in a chair. Use diaphragmatic breathing. Begin at the top of your head. As you inhale, concentrate on and feel the tension in your forehead, as you exhale feel the tension drain away. E.g., while you breathe in mentally say, "forehead" and as you breathe out mentally say "relax" or some other key word. Mentally saying the instructions helps keep you keep focused. Inhale and feel the tension in your temples, and then as you exhale feel the tension drain away from your temples and instruct your temples to relax. Continue with this procedure progressively working down–cheeks and jaw, lips and tongue, neck and throat, shoulders, arms, hands, chest and upper back, stomach, pelvis, thighs, calves, and feet–until your whole body is relaxed. Repeat the exercise three times. A variation is to repeat the forehead relaxation three times, then the temples three times, and so on. Repeat the exercise several times a day.

Note: It is important to feel the tension you are holding in your body and then experience the sensation of tension leaving your body as you relax. It may be helpful to think of this exercise as "a tension or stress meltdown" or as a "Raggedy Ann or Andy" exercise. As you become efficient in relaxing your body, you should be able to do a quick relaxation by going through the procedure once.

APPENDIX 16. Self-Powered Stretches and Exercises for FMS Patients

General Principles

A START LOW–GO SLOW!

Everyday, do what you can but do not over do it. Begin exercising at a comfortable level and gradually increase the duration and intensity of the exercise to coincide with your increased abilities. It is important not to overdo it!

B. WARM UP YOUR MUSCLES

It is helpful to heat up your muscles in a shower, bath, or with hot packs, towels, etc. before stretching. The warmer your muscles are the easier and less painful they are to stretch. Gentle walking will warm up the muscles.

C. FOCUS

Always focus on the muscles you are stretching or working. It is easier to do this when your eyes are closed.

D. BALANCE YOUR MUSCLE WORK

Stretch or work major muscle groups and their opposing muscles. When you work muscles on one side of your body, follow up by working the same muscles on the other side of your body.

E. TROUBLE SHOOTING

1. If an exercise causes pain, reduce the intensity before reducing the frequency.
2. Decrease the time and intensity on bad days but do not overdo it on good days. You should end your exercise sessions feeling you could do a little more.

F. STRETCH, STRETCH, STRETCH!

Stretching is very important. It will loosen up tight, seized, shortened muscles and correct some of the anatomical abnormalities. Muscles that are too short are weaker and more painful than normal when working or exercising. If you work or exercise a tight, short muscle, **before you stretch it out**, it will get tighter, shorter and weaker and more painful. Stretching must be done correctly or it can be painful and counterproductive.

Breathing techniques during stretching are most important.

1. Use your arm, another part of your body, or gravity to help you stretch. Do NOT stretch one muscle on one side of your body with the muscles on the other side!
2. Take the muscle to be stretched to the normal pain free limit.
3. Breathe in and **AS** you breathe out, slowly and gently stretch the muscle a little bit.
4. Hold the muscle at this increased range.
5. **Gradually** build up so you can repeat the stretching cycle within your limits [ideally 3 times].
6. **Never stretch a muscle to the point where you experience pain.**
7. Stretch the opposite muscles and continue to stretch all the groups of muscles you are working on.
8. Your muscles should be easier to stretch, and you should see an increase in the length of your muscles within 7-10 days. If not check your technique.

A few examples of simple effective stretches:

1. Hold the back of your neck at the base of your skull with one hand. Put the other hand on the middle of the top and back of your skull. Hold your neck straight as you stretch you head down at the base of the skull and top of your neck. This will loosen the muscles at the bottom of your skull and top of your neck and improve the blood flow to the brain and help such symptoms as memory and visual changes. The muscles you are stretching are called the suboccipitals.

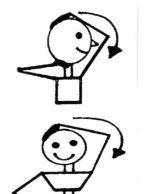

2. Hold a chair or table with one hand to anchor your upper body. Bend your head sideways towards your free hand. Hold the side of your head with the free hand and stretch your head and neck sideways. Repeat on opposite side. This stretch [of the scalenes] will help with the range of sideways motion of your neck and will help with stopping pain, numbness and weakness in your arms, shoulders and neck.

3. Sit in a chair. Using one or both of your hands, push your head back and sideways at a 45° angle. Gradually deepen the stretch using your breathing techniques. This exercise will stretch the sternocleidomastoid muscles [SCM] and help get the head and neck back to their proper place as well as reducing headaches, especially migraines and temporal mandibular joint [TMJ] or jaw problems. [Insert diagram #5.]

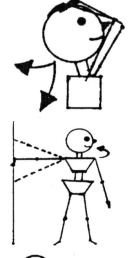

4. Stand in front of a doorway. Reach backwards to grab the door frame. Turn and stretch your shoulders to one side by looking "behind" that shoulder. If you can, do this with your hands in three positions: low, medium, and high. Use your breathing techniques while stretching and repeat on the opposite side. This will stretch your pectoralis muscles and help bring your shoulders backwards to where they belong. This will also help with using your upper body and with lifting and carrying.

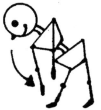

5. Stand with your feet shoulder width apart. Twist your upper body to one side and using your breathing technique, stretch down to touch your foot. Repeat on the opposite side. This exercise will stretch some of the long muscles in your body as well as the quadratus lumborum, which joins the 12th rib to the pelvis.

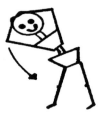

6. Stand with your feet shoulder width apart. Put your hands on top of your head and stretch sideways with your elbow moving towards your knee on that side. Repeat on opposite side. [Insert diagram #8.]

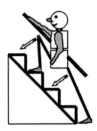

7. Using stairs, put one foot on a stair at a comfortable level, with the other foot stretched behind you and knee straight. Holding onto the stair rail for support, stretch and try to put your knee against a higher stair while you are keeping your head, neck, shoulders, and back **straight** and keeping the sole of your bottom foot flat on the floor. Repeat on other side. This exercise will stretch the quadriceps muscle, the iliopsoas and rectus femoris [muscle at the front of the thigh and pelvis]. This is an important stretch for back, knee, leg and hip pain.

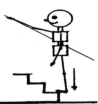

8. Stand on a stair with both your heels over the edge of the stair. Hold on to the stair rail or wall for support. Keep your back straight as you drop your heels to stretch your calves.

9. Lie on your back on the floor. Bend and raise your knees and put the soles of your feet on the floor. Close your eyes and imagine that there is a face of a clock under your buttocks with the hour hand pointing to 12 o'clock. Without changing your actual contact with the floor, use your buttocks and abdominal muscles to point your pelvis to 1 o'clock as you inhale, then relax and return to 12 o'clock as you exhale. Next inhale as you rotate your pelvis towards 2 o'clock and return to 12 o'clock as you exhale. Continue tightening and releasing your muscles as you visualize your pelvis rotating around the clock in this manner. Repeat the exercise in an anti-clockwise direction. This exercise helps loosen up the lower back. Note: Although your buttocks doesn't leave the floor and your pelvis doesn't actually turn to all the numbers of the clock, you are tightening and releasing different sets of muscles in a rotating pattern, thus strengthening and loosening the lower back muscles.

G. STRENGHENING EXERCISES

Exercises must be specific to the patient or muscle group or they can make you worse. The following three exercises are examples of simple but important exercises that should be done daily and will benefit almost everyone with FMS.

1. Tighten up your glutei and abdominal muscles [buttocks and stomach]. These muscles are almost always stretched and inhibited.
2. Keeping your neck straight and tilting your head slightly forward and tucking in your chin, try to push the **bottom** of your neck against your hand, pillow, wall, etc. Do this at night and in the morning. If you tilt your head down slightly, this will also tighten your abdominal muscles as well.
3. Sitting or standing, and using the muscles between your shoulder blades in the middle and lower parts of your back, try to pull your shoulder blades together and down.

H. ENDURANCE EXERCISES

Choose activities you can do within your limits such as walking, or swimming or walking in a warm pool. Do activities at a comfortable pace.

APPENDIX 17. Assessing Occupational Disability

In assessing disability, physicians are called upon to diagnose the patient's condition, and assess the patient's symptoms, functional level and limitations of function, as well as prognosis for recovery and treatment options. Such assessment is based on subjective reports by the patient to physicians as well as objective medical evidence obtained through assessment and diagnostic testing. As third parties are likely to review the complete records of physicians, it is imperative that the physicians maintain detailed, legible and comprehensive notes of the patient's history and clinical determinations made on a contemporaneous basis. Care must be taken to avoid frivolous or off-hand remarks within clinical notes as these can be construed negatively and used against the patient. Physicians should also be mindful not to deviate from their specialty areas and should ensure that the patient is referred to relevant specialists.

In the context of private insurance policies, disability is defined by the degree to which there are limitations on the patient's ability to work, either in their own job or any job for which they are reasonably qualified by way of education, training and experience. With respect to Canada Pension Plan disability benefits, a person is deemed disabled and entitled to benefits when s/he is determined to have a severe and prolonged physical or mental disability by prescribed criteria. A disability is severe if by reason of the disability, the person is incapable of regularly pursuing any substantially gainful occupation. A disability is prolonged only if it is determined in a prescribed manner that the disability is likely to be long continued and of indefinite duration, or is likely to result in death.

A. REQUIREMENTS OF THE OCCUPATIONAL DISABILITY ASSESSMENT

From a medical-legal perspective, assessing occupational disability requires the physician to

1. **Assess symptoms of a patient's disability:** to diagnose the condition, and most importantly to assess the duties of a person's employment and the activities of daily living. The physician is required to give a detailed and comprehensive explanation of how a person's symptoms/condition impose specific functional limitations on the person's ability to engage in the duties of his/her specific job, or in any job for which the person is reasonably qualified by way of education, training and experience, and which would enable the person to earn an income commensurate with that of their present job. Such an assessment should be made in the physician's clinical notes regularly, as these are the source on which third part insurers will rely most heavily.

2. **Assess prognosis:** with respect to a person's anticipated recovery and future employability, as well as the appropriateness of rehabilitative measures. Care must be taken not to set specific deadlines or targets which cannot be met by a patient, as a patient's inability to meet a specific target as prognosed by the physician could be interpreted as malingering on the patient's part, rather than delayed recovery due to the patient's ongoing medical condition.

3. **Assess rehabilitative potential:** As the treating physician is in the best position to assess the patient's ongoing condition, treatment and recovery, s/he should direct and coordinate any rehabilitation efforts and other efforts to return the patient to gainful employment. Vocational rehabilitation service providers may be of assistance in this regard, but their opinions and proposals should never supplant those of the treating physician, who is most directly involved in and responsible for the patient's care and well being.

4. **Provide medical opinion:** as to whether the patient's condition necessitates that s/he remains off work in order to effectuate a cure and/or prevent continued deterioration of the patient's condition. With respect to the impact of disability on the patient's functional limitation of employment, the physician will be required to provide a comprehensive opinion, substantiated by detailed subjective and objective evidence.

B. MEDICAL DOCUMENTATION OF ASSESSMENT OF PERSON'S OCCUPATIONAL DISABILITY

Documentation of the severity of symptoms and disability as a part of ongoing care is essential. The family/attending physician is in the best position to be able to directly ascertain the severity of the patient's symptoms and impact on their ability to function. Reviewing the patient's questionnaires can assist in assessing the impact of the symptoms on the patient's life. They can be roughly graded in the Activities of Daily Living [ADL], which are those activities directly needed for self-care such as bathing, dressing, toileting, feeding, getting in and out of bed/chairs, and walking. They will also impact on the Instrumental Activities of Daily Living [IADL] which directly support the ADL such as meal preparation, shopping, housework, money management, telephone use, and traveling outside the house.

1. **Medical history:** It is important to document the total illness burden on the patient, not just that of the primary diagnosis.
   a. assessment by a specialist conversant with FMS
   b. diagnosis
   c. abnormal laboratory and imaging findings
   d. other objective physiological findings such as orthostatic intolerance and sleep abnormalities
   e. severity of symptoms and their impact on the patients' ability to function in their lifeworld
   f. duration of illness
   g. response to various treatments tried

2. **Questionnaires, scales, and patient's diaries:** As FMS is a syndrome with a recognizable pain pattern, it can be viewed as a coherent entity. It is helpful to have the patient complete a number of questionnaires on their first visit and then periodically so that symptoms and impairments are assessed from many angles. These questionnaires and scales are helpful references in monitoring the patient's status and progress. The following instruments can be used for validation:
   a. **Symptom Severity and Hierarchy Profile [SSHP]:** [Appendix 6] It is helpful to have the patient fill out the symptom severity and hierarchy chart at the initial visit and every six months or so. The scale ranks five common symptoms in order of severity and indicates the severity of each symptom as being absent, mild, moderate, or severe.
   b. **Pain Visual Analog Scale [Pain VAS] and Body Pain Diagram:** [Appendix 7] This is a quick reference that identifies the type, location, and severity of pain the patient experiences.
   c. **Sleep Profile [SP]:** [Appendix 8] The quality and quantity of sleep is an important factor in the patient's ability to function in their daily activities. Having the patient periodically complete the one-week sleep chart and questionnaire assists in identifying and monitoring the difficulties they are having with sleep.
   e. **Fibromyalgia Impact Questionnaire [FIQ]:** [Appendix 9] This instrument is designed to measure components of the health status that are believed to be most affected by FMS.
   f. **Modified Health Assessment Questionnaire [MHAQ]:** This questionnaire also addresses the patient's ability to function in daily activities.
   g. **Daily Activities/Functional Capacity Scale:** Have the patient keep a diary of all his/her daily activities and rest periods for a one-week interval. This should include the timing and duration of the activities as well as a rough quantification, such as specifying type of housework performed, or walking speed and distance. Aggravators should be noted. Patients should rank their functional level on a visual analog scale of 1[totally bedridden] to 10 [functioning normally and feeling energetic] each day during the week. This will help identify cumulative effects, symptom interaction, variance in symptom severity and impact, and long range reactive exacerbation. Encourage the patient to become aware of the relationship between activities and/or activity duration that aggravate her/his symptoms, and then use that knowledge to pace him/herself accordingly.

3. **Other Documentation**
   a. **Computer Science and Application [CSA™] Actigraph:** In cases that need further documentation, a combination of a self-reporting scale and a CSA Actigraph is helpful. This small device is a motion detector that is capable of measuring the frequency and intensity of activity and recording values at 1-minute intervals through the day and night for up to twenty-two [22] consecutive days, thus capturing the dynamics and variability of symptoms (423). The intensity, duration of activity peaks and duration of following rest periods may be compared to those of controls as indicated in van der Werf et al. (424).
   b. **sEMG and qEEG:** These tests usually show abnormalities in FMS patients. They are expensive and not covered by provincial health plans.

4. **Prognosis:** The report should include an estimate of the patient's prognosis. [See Epidemiology, B. Natural History of FMS]

5. **Functional Limitations and Restrictions, and Rehabilitative Potential:** The report should indicate the patient's functional limitations and how the patient's impairments affect his/her ability to do ADL, IADL, function in a rehabilitative program and do work activities.
   a. **Functional limitations and restrictions:** The ability of the patient to participate and function adequately in rehabilitation programs should be assessed over the long term with attention also paid to long range cumulative effects after time spent in the program and the reactivation of symptoms. Disability can occur in the physical, cognitive and emotional realms, in various ratios of interaction and impairment. Attention should be given to:

- **Effects of chronic symptoms:** Chronic pain, fatigue and errors in processing and organizing cognitive experiences have a negative impact on the patient's ability to be competitive in the work force (425-428). They affect the patient's ability to concentrate. Tasks that are tolerated for short periods of time may become aggravators when the task is prolonged (429). Many patients have intolerance for prolonged standing, sitting or doing repetitive tasks. Stress and uncomfortable climatic conditions may significantly aggravate the patient's symptoms.
- **Lack of endurance due to physical and/or mental fatigue:** The patient may have profound worsening of symptoms with previously tolerated amounts of physical and mental activity and develop delayed reactive symptoms.
- **Impaired neurocognitive functions:** The effects of physical fatigue are often amplified by associated loss of mental sharpness as exhibited in poor concentration, difficulty making and consolidating memories, an inability to organize tasks and increased time necessary to accomplish a task, as well as emotional disturbances reactive to the impairment. Loss of short-term memory decreases the efficiency of activity as intentions are started and forgotten and much effort is spent in locating lost articles and they need to constantly reorganize interrupted activities.
- **Unpredictability of symptom dynamics:** Other major sources of work disability in FMS are the lack of endurance, the unpredictable symptom dynamics on a day by day and even an hour to hour basis, and the presence of delayed reactive fatigue and pain and cognitive dysfunction. It usually takes a patient much longer to get going in the morning and many need frequent rests throughout the day. This prevents afflicted patients from taking on regularly scheduled activities, such as are typically required for work-related activities and necessary in the competitive work force.
- **Cumulative effects:** Assess ability to do typical repetitive actions as to duration and to the cumulative effects on fatigue levels over a longer stretch of time.

b. **Assessment by Vocational Rehabilitation Providers:** Assessment by an occupational specialist or a certified occupational therapist [OT] who is knowledgeable about FMS, and experienced in evaluating disability may be helpful but the treating physician should direct and coordinate any rehabilitation efforts.

- **In home assessment:** An OT can provide valuable contextual information about daily function at home [e.g., self care, maintenance of home, endurance, etc.] Level of function at home has direct implications for level of function in the workplace, since employment is a 24-hour issue. Occupational Therapists can also assist the patient with energy conservation principles and in pacing their activities.
- **Workplace assessment:** A workplace assessment provides specific information about physical, mental, emotional, social and environmental job demands. Assessment should be conducted on the job site if possible. Each job should be assessed for aggravators. Many jobs can be adapted for the worker by improving ergonomics, varying job tasks and positions, and with flexibility in scheduling if employer cooperation can be obtained.

c. **Rehabilitation Potential:** The treating physician is most involved in and responsible for the ongoing care and well-being of the patient. The patient's medical management must be optimized prior to the introduction of any rehabilitation program. The treating physician should direct and coordinate treatment and rehabilitation efforts. Rehabilitation personnel must be knowledgeable about FMS. The pathophysiology of FMS must be respected and reflected in the program. Rehabilitation programs must be individualized and accommodate for the patient's total illness burden as well as the day to day variation and fluctuation of the patient's symptom and activity boundaries. The patient must have autonomy over the complexity, duration, and pace of the program. The attending physician should ensure that the patient's symptoms are monitored frequently to observe cumulative effects. Work hardening programs which do not reflect or respect the pathophysiology of FMS and/or autonomy of the patient are not appropriate for the FMS patient and will worsen the patient's symptoms and medical condition.

6. **Provide Medical Opinion:** The information gained through ongoing assessments, scales and questionnaires, patient diaries, etc. equips the attending physician to assess whether the patient is ready for a rehabilitation program, a slow return to work, or is disabled and unable to work due to severity of symptoms. The attending physician should determine whether the patient's medical management is optimized and the illness is sufficiently under control so that the danger of aggravating the patient's symptoms and worsening his/her medical condition during such programs is minimized. It is the responsibility of the attending physician, who is ultimately responsible for the well-being and long-term care of his/her patient, to decide whether such programs are appropriate for the individual patient.

APPENDIX 18. Workplace Aggravators

A wide range of physical and cognitive activities can cause pain, and physical and cognitive fatigue in the FMS patient. When assessing a patient's ability to work, it may be helpful to consider the following common aggravators [adapted from (429)]:

- Prolonged sitting
- Prolonged writing
- Prolonged deskwork or handwork
- Prolonged telephone use
- Prolonged bending over work surface or awkward positioning
- Prolonged standing, walking, or stairs
- Prolonged driving
- Unsupported extension of arms
- Activities that require reaching overhead
- Repeated moving and lifting
- Heavy lifting or carrying
- House cleaning
- Walking more than tolerated distance
- Computer work
- Numerical calculations
- Multi-tasking
- Activities that require remembering what was read or recent events-time sequences
- Fast paced and complex work surroundings, tight deadlines
- Sensory overload: light, sound, odors, motion and confusion
- Change in work hours: e.g., shift work, early hours, long hours, no breaks, jet lag
- Stress
- Environmental factors: e.g., cold, heat, air quality–pollutants, chemicals

APPENDIX 19. Tests that May Be Used Inappropriately in Assessments of FMS

The tests commonly being used to assess the physical capabilities and sincerity of effort of FMS patients are often interpreted inappropriately, as they do not adequately consider the severity and fluctuation of symptoms or the activity level over an extended time frame.

1. **American Medical Association Guide for the Evaluation of Permanent Impairment:** It is futile to use the *American Medical Association Guide for the Evaluation of Permanent Impairment* as it relies on measurements of range of motion and strength to determine total person impairment. The functional disability in FMS is *three dimensional*—the third dimension being time—that is, the patient is unable to sustain repetitive activity (191).

2. **Functional Capacity Evaluations [FCE]** may not reflect the severity and complexity of the illness, nor do they usually assess cognitive fatigue and dysfunction. They are usually one-stop assessments and lack reliable objective methods for determining subject participation [sincerity of effort] (430). When the patient is not able to perform at normal and expected levels, a judgment is made of their sincerity of effort, which may have implications concerning malingering. Since sincerity of effort is a subjective interpretation of the observer and since reliability standards are set on normal subjects, such judgments should not be overemphasized. The performance in the limited, uncharacteristic, and artificial situation of a FCE does not indicate the patient's endurance for a full workday schedule in her/his natural work environment (423) nor does it measure the interaction between physical and cognitive impairments, nor accurately assess when and how activity fluctuations are related to fatigue and/or variable pain levels. One often does not see the full extent of muscle and cognitive fatigue reaction to physical or mental exertion until the day following testing or the pain, fatigue and/or confusion that may be cumulatively increased by activities continued over longer periods of time.

3. **MMPI:** The MMPI was designed to assess the personality status of healthy and psychiatrically ill people. It is seldom useful for patients with FMS. This and similar instruments may be rendered inaccurate by 'confounding' as they do not consider that symptoms such as fatigue, poor sleep, headaches, dizziness, feeling weak, etc. may be due to biological disorders (431). Not only are these symptoms scored as psychiatric symptoms, but also approximately 40 percent of the items are scored more than once as they appear on more than one scale building a bias towards a "neurotic" score (432). Without taking organically caused physical symptoms into account, the interpretation becomes misleading and erroneous.

4. **Waddell's Signs:** were originally used to identify patients with more severe spine disorders but are presently incorrectly interpreted to imply 'non organic' or psychological impairment. The authors of the original data published a clarification that they are not a test of credibility or veracity and cautioned against the misuse of these signs, which has been rampant in disability assessments (433).

APPENDIX 20. Authors' Affiliations and Acknowledgments

Authors' Affiliations

<u>Consensus Panel</u>
Anil Kumar Jain, BSc, MD: Ottawa Hospital, Ottawa, ON, Canada

Bruce M. Carruthers, MD, CM, FRCP[C]: Specialist in Internal Medicine, Saanichton, BC, Canada

I. Jon Russell, MD, PhD, FACR: Associate Professor of Medicine, Division of Clinical Immunology; Director, University Clinical Research Center, University of Texas Health Science Center, San Antonio, Texas, USA; Editor, *Journal of Musculoskeletal Pain*; International Pain Consultant to Pain Research & Management, *The Journal of the Canadian Pain Society*, London, ON; Editorial Board of *Pain Watch*; Honorary Board Member of the Lupus Foundation of America

Thomas J. Romano, MD, PhD, FACP, FACR: Diplomat and President of the Board of Directors of the American Academy of Pain Management; Editorial Board and Columnist, *Journal of Musculoskeletal Pain*; Advisory Panel, Health Points/TyH Publications; East Ohio Regional Hospital, Martins Ferry, Ohio, USA

Dan S. Heffez, MD, FRCS: President, Heffez Neurosurgical Associates S.C.; and Associate Professor of Neurosurgery, Rush Medical College, Chicago, Illinois, USA

Daniel G. Malone, MD: Associate Professor of Medicine, University of Wisconsin, Wisconsin, USA

Donald G. Seibel, BSc [Med], MD, CAFCI: Medical Director, Mayfield Pain and Musculoskeletal Clinic, Edmonton, AB, Canada

Stephen R. Barron, MD, CCFP, FCFP: Clinical Assistant Professor, Department of Family Practice, Faculty of Medicine, University of British Columbia; Medical Staff, Royal Columbian Hospital, New Westminster, BC, Canada

C. C. Stuart Donaldson, PhD: Director, Myosymmetries, Calgary, AB, Canada

James V. Dunne, MB, FRCP[C]: Clinical Assistant Professor, Department of Medicine, University of British Columbia; Vancouver General and St. Paul's Hospitals, Vancouver, BC, Canada

Emerson Gingrich, MD, CCFP[C]: Family practice, retired, Calgary, AB, Canada

Frances Y.-K. Leung, BSc, MD, FRCP[C]: Clinical Lecturer, Faculty of Medicine, University of Toronto; Department of Rheumatology, Sunnybrook and Women's College Health Science Centre; Department of Medicine, Saute Area Hospitals, ON, Canada

David Saul, MD, CCFP[C]: Private practice, North York, ON, Canada

<u>Consensus Coordinator:</u>
Marjorie I. van de Sande, BEd, Grad Dip Ed: Director of Education, National ME/FM Action Network, Canada

Author Contribution

Consensus Panel: *Anil Kumar Jain and Bruce M. Carruthers [collaborated as co-editors on the position paper developed for Health Canada] Stephen R. Barron, C. C. Stuart Donaldson, James V. Dunne, Emerson Gingrich, Daniel S. Heffez, Frances Y.-K. Leung, Daniel G. Malone, Thomas J. Romano, I. Jon Russell, David Saul, Donald G. Seibel [actively participated in the review process and in the development of the consensus document].*
Consensus Coordinator: *Marjorie I. van de Sande contributed to and compiled the consensus document.*

All authors gave approval to the final document.

Acknowledgements

Lydia Neilson, President and CEO, and the **National ME/FM Action Network** for spearheading the drive for the development of a clinical case definition, and diagnostic and treatment protocols for FMS.

Health Canada, for establishing the "Terms of Reference," and the selection of the Expert Consensus Panel.

Crystaal, for sponsoring the Expert Consensus Panel Workshop in Toronto, ON, Canada.

Kim Dupree Jones, RNC, PhD, FNP, exercise physiologist, for her input in the exercise/treatment section.

Kerry Ellison, OT [non-practicing], for her input in the patient management/treatment section, and the assessing disability appendix.

Hugh Scher, LLP, for his input in the assessing disability appendix.

Correspondence to: *Dr. Anil Kumar Jain, 118, 1025 Grenon Avenue, Ottawa, ON K2B 8S5, Canada. Fax: [613] 596-3212.*
E-mail to Dr. Bruce M. Carruthers: **(bcarruth@telus.net)**

Authors' Affiliations

Consensus Panel:
Anil Kumar Jain, BSc, MD: Ottawa Hospital, Ottawa, ON, Canada.
    Address: 118, 1025 Grenon Avenue, Ottawa, ON, K2B 8S5, Canada. Fax: [613] 596-3212, no e-mail.

Bruce M. Carruthers, MD, CM, FRCP[C]: Specialist in Internal Medicine.
    Address: Suite 308, 7840 Lochside Drive, Saanichton, BC, V8M 2B9, Canada. Fax: [250] 652-6663 (*bcarruth@telus.net*)

Stephen R. Barron, MD, CCFP, FCFP: Clinical Assistant Professor, Department of Family Practice, Faculty of Medicine, University of British Columbia; Medical Staff, Royal Columbian Hospital, New Westminster, BC, Canada.
    Address: #1, 2185 Wilson Avenue, Port Coquitlam, BC, V3C 6C1, Canada. Fax: [604] 942-7058 (*sbarron@interchange.ubc.ca*)

C. C. Stuart Donaldson, PhD: Director, Myosymmetries, Calgary, AB, Canada.
    Address: 300, 290 Midpark Way SE, Calgary, AB, T2X 1P1, Canada. Fax: [403] 225-2389 (*myo@telus.net*)

James V. Dunne, MB, FRCP[C]: Clinical Assistant Professor, Department of Medicine, University of British Columbia; Vancouver General and St. Paul's Hospitals, Vancouver, BC, Canada.
    Address: 700 West 57 Avenue, Vancouver, BC, V6P 1S1. Fax [604] 321-7833, (*jdunne@vanhosp.bc.ca*)

Emerson Gingrich, MD, CCFP[C]: Family practice, retired, Calgary, AB, Canada.
    Address: C202, 1919 University Drive N.W., Calgary, T2N 4K5. Phone: [403] 650-5406. [No fax or e-mail]

Dan S. Heffez, MD, FRCS: President, Heffez Neurosurgical Associates S.C.; and Associate Professor of Neurosurgery, Rush Medical College, Chicago, Illinois, USA.
    Address: 2900 North Lake Shore Drive, Suite 1201, Chicago, Illinois 60657, USA. Fax: [773] 281-4472, (*dheffez@sbcglobal.net*)

Frances Y.-K. Leung, BSc, MD, FRCP[C]: Clinical Lecturer, Faculty of Medicine, University of Toronto; Department of Rheumatology, Sunnybrook and Women's College Health Science Centre; Department of Medicine, Saute Area Hospitals, ON, Canada.
    Address: Suite 202, 855 Broadview Avenue, Toronto, ON, M4K 3Z1, Canada. Fax [416] 462-1220 (*ykrheum@yahoo.com*)

Daniel G. Malone, MD: Associate Professor of Medicine, University of Wisconsin, Wisconsin, USA.
  Address: University of Wisconsin, 600 Highland Avenue, Room H6-363, Madison, WI 53792-3244 USA.
  Fax: [608] 263-9660, (*dgm@medicine.wisc.edu*)

Thomas J. Romano, MD, PhD, FACP, FACR: Diplomat and President of the Board of Directors of the American Academy of Pain Management; Editorial Board and Columnist, *Journal of Musculoskeletal Pain*; Advisory Panel, Health Points/TyH Publications; East Ohio Regional Hospital, Martins Ferry, Ohio.
  Address: 205 North 5th Street, Martins Ferry, OH 43935 USA. Fax: [740] 633-2016, (*crazydoc49@aol.com*)

I. Jon Russell, MD, PhD, FACR: Associate Professor of Medicine, Division of Clinical Immunology; Director, University Clinical Research Center, University of Texas Health Science Center, San Antonio, Texas, USA.; Editor, *Journal of Musculoskeletal Pain*; International Pain Consultant to Pain Research & Management, *The Journal of the Canadian Pain Society*, London, ON; Editorial Board of *Pain Watch*; Honorary Board Member of the Lupus Foundation of America.
  Address: Department of Medicine, Mail Code 7868, UTHSCSA, 7703 Floyd Curl Drive, San Antonio, TX, 78229-3900 USA. Fax [210] 567-6669 (*russell@uthscsa.edu*)

David Saul, MD, CCFP[C]: Private practice, North York, ON, Canada.
  Address: 80 Finch Avenue West, North York, ON, M2N 2H4, Canada. Fax: [416] 221-5599 (*drdavidsaul@rogers.com*)

Donald G. Seibel, BSc [Med], MD, CAFCI: Medical Director, Mayfield Pain and Musculoskeletal Clinic, Edmonton, AB, Canada.
  Address: Mayfield Pain & Musculoskeletal Clinic, 11054–156 Street, Edmonton, AB, T5P 4M8, Canada. Fax: [780] 487-4204 (*drseibel@telusplanet.net*)

Consensus Coordinator:
Marjorie I. van de Sande, BEd, Grad Dip Ed: Director of Education, National ME/FM Action Network, Canada
  Address: 151 Arbour Ridge Circle N.W., Calgary, AB, T3G 3V9, Canada. Phone & Fax: [403] 547-8799s (*mvandes@shaw.ca*)

Proposed Study to Develop and Validate a Clinical Case Definition for the Fibromyalgia Syndrome Applicable to the Clinical Practice Setting

I. Jon Russell

The 1990 American College of Rheumatology [ACR] Criteria (1) for the Classification of the fibromyalgia syndrome [FMS] were intended principally to facilitate uniform screening of patients to enter FMS research studies. They have been dramatically fruitful in that respect since the numbers of research studies on the subject of FMS subsequently increased from under 20 published per year to over 200 per year and climbing [see Figure 1]. Clearly, these criteria met a perceived need in the medical community and have opened up the FMS for exploration by modern clinical, imaging, and laboratory methodologies.

There is little doubt that the designers of these criteria were aware of the probability that these criteria would soon be applied in the clinic, particularly if they were successful in the research arena. In fact, this pattern would seem to have been the modus operandi of the ACR with regard to many of the clinical disorders under its clinical umbrella. As a result, there are defined criteria for the diagnosis of osteoarthritis (2), rheumatoid arthritis (3), systemic lupus erythematosus (4), systemic sclerosis (5), and a variety of other conditions listed in the Primer on the Rheumatic Diseases (6).

It is not entirely clear why the FMS came to rest under the "shingle" of the rheumatologist when the current view of FMS's central nervous system pathogenesis seems to better fit the pathogenic profile of a neurologist's practice. One could speculate that early on, there was a perception among referring physicians, and even among perceptive patients, that the

I. Jon Russell, MD, PhD, is Associate Professor of Medicine, Division of Clinical Immunology; Director, University Clinical Research Center, University of Texas Health Science Center, San Antonio, Texas, USA, Editor, *Journal of Musculoskeletal Pain*; International Pain Consultant to Pain Research & Management, *The Journal of the Canadian Pain Society*, London, ON; Editorial Board of *Pain Watch*, Honorary Board Member of the Lupus Foundation of America.

[Haworth co-indexing entry note]: "Proposed Study to Develop and Validate a Clinical Case Definition for the Fibromyalgia Syndrome Applicable to the Clinical Practice Setting." Russell, I. Jon. Co-published simultaneously in *Journal of Musculoskeletal Pain* [The Haworth Medical Press, an imprint of The Haworth Press, Inc.] Vol. 11. No. 4, 2003, pp. 109-111; and: *The Fibromyalgia Syndrome: A Clinical Case Definition for Practitioners* [ed: I. Jon Russell] The Haworth Medical Press, an imprint of The Haworth Press, Inc., 2003, pp. 109-111. Single or multiple copies of this article are available for a fee from The Haworth Document Delivery Service [1-800-HAWORTH, 9:00 a.m. - 5:00 p.m. [EST]. E-mail address: docdelivery@haworthpress.com].

FIGURE 1. Annual publications about the Fibromyalgia Syndrome [FMS]. Notice the sharp rise in publications which accompanies the development lightly antedates the publication of the 1990 American College of Rheumatology criteria for the classification of FMS. It seems likely that the availability of the published criteria has facilitated development and publication of studies thereafter.

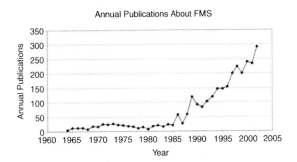

symptoms of body pain, morning stiffness, physical limitation, and emotive consequences resembled many of the other conditions in the rheumatologists' stable. In response, rheumatologists were among the first to take the condition seriously and to apply modern methodology to its examination (7). While some rheumatologists (8,9) now argue that FMS should not be receiving the kind of attention it currently commands, it is naïve to assume that the FMS, with its recognized world-wide distribution, will obediently vanish to satisfy the critics' restrictive view of the "run-away" world around them.

One point (10) is readily conceded. There has been a growing recognition of the need for a validated, clinical case definition that can be used to diagnose and manage FMS in the practices of community physicians. The Canadians have been the first to offer a consensus (11) regarding a clinical case definition that was specifically developed for this purpose. This document represented a clear call to develop and validate a clinical case definition for the purpose of use in clinical practice. On very short notice, *JMP* has recruited two well respected, world-class epidemiologists, with a track record for studying FMS, to offer their opinions regarding the kind of study[ies] needed to develop such a clinical case definition and to validate it for use in community medicine. As a format for their presentations, the following working outline was submitted to both of them. Their ideas are provided in the subsequent Research Ideas documents (12,13). As always for this format, these authors should at least be quoted, and preferably invited to involvement, if any of their ideas are used in future grant proposal or in a manuscript focusing on the concept of a clinical case definition of FMS.

Working Outline:

Title: Suggest a title

Investigators: Who you think would be the critical people in leadership of the study to make it happen and by their credentials in the field give it validity what ever the outcome?

Hypotheses: That some combination of the ACR Criteria and other clinical measures will properly identify FMS in clinical practice. Are there other hypotheses?

Specific Aims: To identify a Clinical Case Definition of FMS for routine use by clinical practitioners. Are there other Specific Aims?

Settings: Types of practices that should be chosen to participate, staff needed such as Delphi, blinded examiner?

Inclusion: Seeking all comers with body pain?, limited to widespread pain, other points, What would be the gold standard?

Sample Size: Numbers of clinical offices, numbers of FMS patients, number of other conditions to include as normal controls, which kinds of disease controls?

Outcomes: Measures to include, primary outcome variables, critical other variables, approaches to identify FMS subgroups, different modes of onset?

Methods: Do you think we are ready to conduct such a study with study subjects answering questions and staff documenting findings directly on the internet so data quality control would be less of an issue than it can be with a multicenter project?

Statistics: Approaches to use?

Cost: Rough estimate of what you think this study would cost and who you think might be interested in funding the study.

REFERENCES

1. Wolfe F, Smythe HA, Yunus MB, Bennett RM, Bombardier C, Goldenberg DL, Tugwell P, Campbell SM, Abeles M, Clark P, Fam AG, Farber SJ, Fiechtner JJ, Franklin CM, Gatter RA, Hamaty D, Lessard J, Lichtbroun AS, Masi AT, McCain GA, Reynolds WJ, Romano TJ, Russell IJ, Sheon RP: The American College of Rheumatology 1990 Criteria for the Classification of Fibromyalgia. Arthritis Rheum 33:160-172, 1990.

2. Altman R, Asch E, Bloch D, Bole G, Borenstein D, Brandt K, Christy W, Cooke TD, Greenwald R, Hochberg M, Howell D, Kaplan D, Koopman W, Longley SI, Mankin H, McShane DJ, Medsger TJ, Meenan R, Mikkelsen W, Moskowitz R, Murphy W, Rothschild B, Segal M, Sokoloff L, Wolfe F: Development of criteria for the classifiction and reporting of osteoarthritis. Arthritis Rheum 29:1039-1049, 1986.

3. Arnett FC, Edworthy SM, Bloch DA, McShane DJ, Fries JF, Cooper NS, Healey LA, Kaplan SR, Liang MH, Luthra HS, Medsger TAJr, Mitchell DM, Neustadt DH, Pinals RS, Schaller JG, Sharp JT, Wilder RL, Hunder GG: The American Rheumatism Association 1987 revised criteria for the classification of rheumatoid arthritis. Arthritis Rheum 31:315-324, 1988.

4. Tan EM, Cohen AS, Fries JF et al.: The 1992 revised criteria for the classification of systemic lupus erythematosus. Arthritis Rheum 25:1271-1277, 1982.

5. Subcommittee for Scleroderma Criteria of the American Rheumatism Association Diagnostic and Therapeutic Criteria Committee: Preliminary criteria for the classification of systemic sclerosis (scleroderma). Arthritis Rheum 23:581-590, 1980.

6. Klippel JH: Primer on the Rheumatic Diseases. 11 Edition, Arthritis Foundation, Atlanta, Georgia, USA, 1997.

7. Russell IJ: Fibromyalgia. In: Bonica's Management of Pain. Edited by JD Loeser. Williams & Wilkins, New York, New York, 2000, pp. 543-559.

8. Ehrlich GE: Pain Is Real; Fibromyalgia Isn't. J Rheumatol 30(8):1666-1667, 2003. (Abstract)

9. Hadler NM: "Fibromyalgia" and the Medicalization of Misery. J Rheumatol 30(8):1668-1670, 2003. (Abstract)

10. Wolfe F: Stop Using the American College of Rheumatology Criteria in the Clinic. J Rheumatol 30 (8):1671-1672, 2003. (Abstract)

11. Jain AK, Carruthers BM, van de Sande MI, Barron SR, Donaldson CCS, Dunne JV, Gingrich E, Heffez DS, Leung, FY-K, Malone DJ, Romano, TJ, Russell IJ, Saul D, Seibel DG: Fibromyalgia syndrome: Canadian clinical working case definition, diagnostic and treatment protocols–A consensus document. J Musculoske Pain 11(4): 3-107, 2003.

12. White KP: Developing and validating a clinical case definition for the fibromyalgia syndrome for use in clinical practice. J Musculoske Pain 11(4):117-118, 2003.

13. Raphael KG: Proposed methods for validation of a clinical case definition of the fibromyalgia syndrome. J Musculoske Pain 11(4):113-115, 2003.

Proposed Methods for Validation of a Clinical Case Definition of the Fibromyalgia Syndrome

Karen G. Raphael

The Canadian Consensus Clinical Working Case Definition (1) proposes an alternative to the 1990 American College of Rheumatology [ACR] criteria (2) for the fibromyalgia syndrome [FMS], stating that the latter was primarily created to standardize research. While the development of the ACR criteria might have been driven initially by the imperative to standardize criteria to allow replication across FMS research studies, any case definition is handicapped as both a research and clinical tool, if it does not adequately reflect the clinical construct; that is, if it does not identify the typical individual identified by expert clinicians as having FMS. From a research perspective, such a definition would be said to lack "content validity."

Delimination from other disorders as part of case definition validation. The initial validation study of the ACR criteria, provided important validity data by showing that the criteria differentiated FMS from other disorders potentially confused with FMS. Delimination from other disorders is a critical validation standard. Nevertheless, a limitation to the sole validation study is that the case sample consisted of individuals who had already been identified as prototypic FMS in tertiary care rheumatology (or even more specialized, high-profile FMS) practices, and the contrast group consisted of patients seen in the same settings for other pain or rheumatological conditions. Would these same ACR criteria work to differentiate between those with FMS and those who regularly engage in a couple of bar fights each month and have, therefore, widespread pain and diffuse tender points over the past three months? Case criteria that may have demonstrated some utility in the rheumatology clinic may have less utility in a primary care setting and little or no utility when applied outside of treatment settings. By adding other potential physiological dysfunctions to the ACR diagnostic criteria, the potential exists for improving delimination between FMS and "non-FMS" in other clinical and community settings. One new study to evaluate the validity of the proposed clinical working case definition might involve a general replication of the initial ACR validation study, but might be conducted in a primary care or even general population setting. Such a study would need to demonstrate that application of the additional clinical signs and symptoms aids differentiation between those with prototypic FMS and those with widespread pain secondary to a diverse group of causes [not just other conditions seen com-

Karen G. Raphael, PhD, is Associate Professor, University of Medicine & Dentistry of New Jersey, 30 Bergen Street ADMC 14004B, Newark, NJ 07107 USA.

[Haworth co-indexing entry note]: "Proposed Methods for Validation of a Clinical Case Definition of the Fibromyalgia Syndrome." Raphael, Karen G. Co-published simultaneously in *Journal of Musculoskeletal Pain* [The Haworth Medical Press, an imprint of The Haworth Press, Inc.] Vol. 11, No. 4, 2003, pp. 113-115; and: *The Fibromyalgia Syndrome: A Clinical Case Definition for Practitioners* [ed: I. Jon Russell] The Haworth Medical Press, an imprint of The Haworth Press, Inc., 2003, pp. 113-115. Single or multiple copies of this article are available for a fee from The Haworth Document Delivery Service [1-800-HAWORTH, 9:00 a.m. - 5:00 p.m. [EST]. E-mail address: docdelivery@haworthpress. com].

http://www.haworthpress.com/web/JMP
© 2003 by The Haworth Press, Inc. All rights reserved.
Digital Object Identifer: 10.1300/J094v11n04_04

monly in rheumatology practices] that are considered to be extraneous to FMS.

Delimination from other disorders is just one standard for validating a case definition. The classic approach to psychiatric syndrome validity (3) provides a model for using longitudinal observation and familial aggregation [and possibly more sophisticated genetics studies] as validation standards for diagnostic criteria developed for complex syndromes.

For example, is the clinical course and prognosis for those who present with 10 tender points different than the clinical course and prognosis for those who present with 11 or more tender points? The validation of the tender point cut-point of 11, to date, has only been demonstrated by showing that it best differentiated FMS patients from controls. However, if clinical outcome is ultimately the same for those with 10 versus 11 tender point counts, validation for the existing cut point will not have been firmly established. We can extend this argument to the additional proposed clinical criteria. Specifically, only a subset of patients meeting ACR criteria manifest neurological or neurocognitive difficulties; if these addition difficulties do not help predict the patient's probable onset factors, longitudinal course, treatment-responsiveness, or overall prognosis, they lack predictive clinical utility and probably should not be added to the case definition.

Homogeneity of longitudinal course as part of case definition validation. If individuals meeting a set of diagnostic criteria proceed along a prototypic illness trajectory, the diagnostic standards are valid in that they have heuristic value for predicting long-term prognosis. Although several studies of long-term prognosis in selected clinical samples with FMS have been conducted, only one (4) was community-based. It focused on the effects of labeling those with chronic widespread pain with "fibromyalgia" on 36-month outcome, but did not attempt to address the issue of diagnostic validity. Moreover, unless those individuals followed longitudinally had FMS symptoms of recent onset, inferences about the natural history of FMS are impossible.

Thus, one study that could provide validation data for the working case definition would involve examination of the longitudinal symptom course of those who meet some [but not all] as well as those who meet all of the proposed clinical case criteria. Ideally, this natural history method of syndrome validation would recruit such individuals from the general community, and participants would have recent onset of their symptoms. Again, recruitment from general community samples is important, as selective pathways into treatment may cause a disabled individual with FMS, who seeks or receives no care, to have a different symptom profile from a disabled individual with FMS who has the resources to be treated in a highly specialized rheumatology practice.

Undertaking such studies would likely require federal [e.g., NIH] support. For example, it might involve a two-stage sampling procedure [i.e., large-sample telephone screening of a random sample of community residents in a defined geographic area, followed by a comprehensive in-person examination] to identify groups of community residents who:

1. meet current ACR criteria for FMS, or
2. meet a less stringent definition of FMS [e.g., nine or ten tender points, three rather than four quadrant pain], or
3. meet ACR criteria for FMS, *plus* the various, additional, proposed signs and symptoms.

For each sample, one would select only those with recent onset [< 6 months] symptoms, a methodological requirement for reasonable causal inference. Such a strategy could only be implemented by screening a large community sample. We could then follow these initial subjects closely over the course of at least four years, conducting comprehensive re-examinations and assessments of pain and disability every six months.

Familial aggregation as part of case definition validation. One of the classic standards for complex syndrome validation is familial aggregation. Numerous studies now demonstrate familial aggregation of FMS, using 1990 ACR criteria. Additional studies, showing that the extent of familial aggregation is, at best, improved or, at worst, unchanged, when adding additional clinical criteria, would provide evidence of clinical case definition validation. More sophisticated genetics studies of FMS have suggested that genetic polymorphisms in serotonin-related genes may be involved. Similar studies validating these findings, but applying an expanded clinical case definition, would provide the strongest evidence for a shared, genetically mediated pathogenesis for both compulsory and proposed, additional clinical signs and symptoms.

In summary, validation of the Canadian Clinical Working Case Definition of FMS cannot be accomplished in a single study. It would require a convergence of evidence from multiple studies addressing the utility of the clinical case definition to delimit FMS from other conditions, to predict longitudinal course, and to identify a syndrome with shared, genetically mediated risk factors.

REFERENCES

1. Jain AK, Carruthers BM, van de Sande MI, Barron SR, Donaldson CCS, Dunne JV, Gingrich E, Heffez DS, Leung FY-K, Malone DJ, Romano TJ, Russell IJ, Saul D, Seibel DG: Fibromyalgia syndrome: Canadian clinician working case definition, diagnostic and treatment protocols–A consensus document. J Musculoske Pain 11(4):3-107, 2003.

2. Wolfe F, Smythe HA, Yunus MB, Bennett RM, Bombardier C, Goldenberg DL, Tugwell P, Campbell SM, Abeles M, Clark P, Fam AG, Farber SJ, Fiechtner JJ, Franklin CM, Gatter RA, Hamaty D, Lessard J, Lichtbroun AS, Masi AT, McCain GA, Reynolds WJ, Romano TJ, Russell IJ, Sheon RP: The American College of Rheumatology 1990 Criteria for the Classification of Fibromyalgia. Arthritis Rheum 33:160-172, 1990.

3. Robins E, Guze SB: Establishment of diagnostic validity in psychiatric illness: its application to schizophrenia. Am J Psychiatry 126:983-987, 1970.

4. White KP, Nielson WR, Harth M, Ostbye T, Speechley M: Does the label "fibromyalgia" alter health status, function, and health service utilization? A prospective, within-group comparison in a community cohort of adults with chronic widespread pain. Arthritis Rheum 47:260-265, 2002.

Developing and Validating a Clinical Case Definition for the Fibromyalgia Syndrome for Use in Clinical Practice

Kevin P. White

What follows is a very limited summary of the steps that would be required to examine any clinical case definition for the fibromyalgia syndrome [FMS]. Before actually initiating such a project, I would meet with some of my past collaborators, who have included clinical and population epidemiologists, rheumatologists, and statisticians. Participation by all of these fields would be necessary to undertake what I would consider to be a monumentous, but hugely valuable undertaking.

The development and validation of a clinically useful case definition for the fibromyalgia syndrome [FMS] would necessarliy be a multi-stage process. It would require large numbers of subjects with FMS and a similarly large number of subjects without FMS. Such a study would have to be multi-centered, requiring participation from numerous investigators with expertise in clinical and population epidemiology, rheumatology and biostatistics.

The working definition provided in the Canadian Consensus (1) manuscript could be viewed as a starting point. A panel of clinical investigators would begin by reviewing all the components of the proposed case definition, trying to eliminate duplication so that a reasonably limited number of criteria can be evaluated.

Once content validity [that the criteria being evaluated seem reasonable to assess the disorder of interest] has been determined, the next step should be cluster analysis. This would help to avoid the problem of tautology[1] that often has been a concern with the 1990 ACR criteria (2) Cluster analysis should be performed at multiple sites using a large number of adults who have nothing in common other than the complaint of chronic, widespread pain [CWP]. Recruiting such subjects, given the desire to create a case definition that might be useful not only in tertiary care, but also in primary and secondary care settings, would best be performed at the primary care level [family practice and general medicine clinics]. Adults attending a representative number of geographically dispersed clinics should be screened using a cientifically validated screening instrument for FMS such as the London Fibromyalgia Epidemiology Study Screening Questionnaire [LFESSQ]. Sample size estimation would need to consider the number of potential criteria being assessed.[2]

Eligible subjects who agree to participate should then complete a health questionnaire asking about all of the symptoms and signs contained within the proposed case definition. This questionnaire first should have been validated for content and tested for test-retest reliability on a smaller, representative sample of adults with FMS and a similar number of adult normal controls and adults with other painful conditions other than FMS, by having the same

Kevin P. White, MD, PhD, Rheumatology and Epidemiology, 310-266 Oxford Street East, London, Ontario N6A 1V1.

[Haworth co-indexing entry note]: "Developing and Validating a Clinical Case Definition for the Fibromyalgia Syndrome for Use in Clinical Practice." White, Kevin P. Co-published simultaneously in *Journal of Musculoskeletal Pain* [The Haworth Medical Press, an imprint of The Haworth Press, Inc.] Vol. 11, No. 4, 2003, pp. 117-118; and: *The Fibromyalgia Syndrome: A Clinical Case Definition for Practitioners* [ed: I. Jon Russell] The Haworth Medical Press, an imprint of The Haworth Press, Inc., 2003, pp. 117-118. Single or multiple copies of this article are available for a fee from The Haworth Document Delivery Service [1-800-HAWORTH, 9:00 a.m. - 5:00 p.m. [EST]. E-mail address: docdelivery@ haworthpress.com].

subjects complete the same questionnaire on two occasions, one week apart, to determine agreement between first and second responses to each item. A test-retest reliability value of at least 90% should be considered a minimum requirement for every item on the questionnaire.

Then each of the eligible subjects in the cluster analysis study should be examined by two to three examiners blinded both to pre-existing diagnoses and to the findings and conclusions of earlier examiners. At each site, examiners should have been pre-tested to determine intra- and inter-observer variability for each physical test.

All data collected then would be entered into detailed cluster analysis to determine clusters of patients and the determinants of each cluster. This analysis could lead to identification of more than one FMS-like cluster. Hence, the results would need to go back to the initial content validation committee to group potential clusters and to provide a final, testable case definition for fibromyalgia. An advantage of this ap proach is that investigators may be able to identify FMS subgroups which may exhibit different features of natural history, different associations with co-morbid conditions, different risk factors, different laboratory abnormalities, and different responses to treatment.

Validation of this new case definition then would require examination of:

1. test-retest-reliability;
2. intra- and inter-observer variability in clinics different from those already involved in the cluster analysis;
3. sensitivity; and
4. specificity assessments.

Since there is no 'gold standard' by which to confirm FMS, sensitivity and specificity

should be tested by re-examining subjects previously determined to fall within a given cluster, in a different clinic with different blinded examiners.

Obviously, this is not a single study. It is a stepwise research program that will require several years of diligent investigation, supported by major research funding. A huge advantage of this research, however, is that it may lead us to a much improved understanding of FMS and related conditions, including understanding of risk factors, comorbidity, causes of disease, natural history, and prognosis.

NOTES

1. Critics claim that the process of selecting individuals thought to have FMS and then developing criteria to distinguish them from individuals not thought to have FMS in inherently circular and, hence, flawed.

2. Hence the reason to avoid duplication.

REFERENCES

1. Jain AK, Carruthers BM, van de Sande MI, Barron SR, Donaldson CCS, Dunne JV, Gingrich JV, Gingrich E, Heffez DS, Leung FY-K, Malone DJ, Romano TJ, Russell IJ, Saul D, Seibel DG: Fibromyalgia syndrome: Canadian clinical working case definition, diagnostic and treatment protocols–A consensus document. J Musculoske pain 11(4):3-107, 2003.

2. Wolfe F, Smythe HA, Yunus MB, Bennett RM, Bombardier C, Goldenberg DL, Tugwell P, Campbell SM, Abeles M, Clark P, Fam AG, Farber SJ, Fiechtner JJ, Franklin CM, Gatter RA, Hamaty D, Lessard J, Lichtbroun AS, Masi AT, McCain GA, Reynolds WJ, Romano TJ, Russell IJ, Sheon RP: The American College of Rheumatology 1990 Criteria for the Classification of Fibromyalgia. Arthritis Rheum 33:160-172, 1990.

Index